MANAGED CARE
AND THE
TREATMENT
OF
CHRONIC
ILLNESS

MANAGED CARE AND THE TREATMENT OF CHRONIC ILLNESS

Jon B. Christianson
University of Minnesota

Aylin Altan Riedel
Ingenix Pharmaceutical Services

David J. Abelson
Park Nicollet Clinic and Methodist Hospital, St. Louis Park, Minnesota

Richard L. Hamer
Interstudy Publications

David J. Knutson
Park Nicollet Institute for Research and Education

Ruth A. Taylor
University of Minnesota

Sage Publications
International Educational and Professional Publisher
Thousand Oaks ■ London ■ New Delhi

Copyright © 2001 by Sage Publications, Inc.

All rights reserved. No part of this book may be reproduced or utilized in any form or by any means, electronic or mechanical, including photocopying, recording, or by any information storage and retrieval system, without permission in writing from the publisher.

For information:

Sage Publications, Inc.
2455 Teller Road
Thousand Oaks, California 91320
E-mail: order@sagepub.com

Sage Publications Ltd.
6 Bonhill Street
London EC2A 4PU
United Kingdom

Sage Publications India Pvt. Ltd.
M-32 Market
Greater Kailash I
New Delhi 110 048 India

Printed in the United States of America

Library of Congress Cataloging-in-Publication Data

Christianson, Jon B.
  Managed care and the treatment of chronic illness / by Jon B. Christianson, Aylin Altan Riedel, David J. Abelson.
    p. cm.
  Includes bibliographical references and index.
  ISBN 0-7619-1967-8
  1. Chronically ill—Medical care—United States. 2. Managed care plans (Medical care)—United States. I. Riedel, Aylin Altan. II. Abelson, David. III. Title.
  RA644.6 .C47 2001
  362.1′04258′0973—dc21   2001001025

This book is printed on acid-free paper.

01 02 03 04 05 06 07 7 6 5 4 3 2 1

Acquisition Editor:	Rolf Janke
Editorial Assistant:	Mishelle Gold
Production Editor:	Sanford Robinson
Editorial Assistant:	Kathryn Journey
Typesetter:	Tina Hill
Indexer:	Will Ragsdale
Cover Designer:	Michelle Lee

Contents

Foreword by Edward Wagner	ix
Preface	xv
1. Introduction	**1**
Defining Chronic Illness	3
Defining Managed Care/Managed Care Organizations	5
Organizing the Literature Review and Synthesis	8
Searching for Relevant Literature	10
Appendix: Description of Illnesses	11
2. Chronic Illness and Managed Care:	
What Are the issues?	**21**
People With Chronic Illness	22
The Shift to Managed Care	23
Early Concerns	26
Current Debate	30
Research Issues	35

3. **Individuals With Chronic Illness:**
   MCO Versus Fee-for-Service Comparisons   39
       Discussion   59

4. **The Prevalence of Chronic Illness Management**
   Programs in Managed Care Organizations   65
       Background   66
       Small-Scale Studies   68
       The Wagner et al. Study   70
       The InterStudy Survey   72
       Vendor Products and Chronic Illness "Carve-Outs"   80
       Vendor Products for Use With Multiple Diseases   81
       Vendor Products for Specific Chronic Illnesses   82
       Discussion   86

5. **Use of Administrative and Medical Records Data**
   by MCOs for Chronic Illness Management   89
       Benchmarking   91
       Assessment of Quality of Care   93
       Identification of Opportunities for Improvement   95
       Profiling of Clinics and Providers   97
       Characterization of High-Risk Patients   99
       Simulation of Disease Management Interventions   100
       Summary   103
       Appendix:
           Studies That Use Administrative Claims
           and Medical Records Review to Assess the
           Management of Chronic Illnesses in Managed
           Care Organizations   105

6. **The Effectiveness of Targeted Initiatives**
   in Treating Chronic Illnesses   113
       Some Definitions   116
       Criteria for Study Selection   118
       Overview of Review Process   119
       Diabetes   122
       Asthma   131
       Congestive Heart Failure   138

Cardiovascular Disease	147
Arthritis	155
Overall Summary and Conclusions	166
Appendix A:	
Literature Describing Diabetes Management Programs in Managed Care Organizations	172
Appendix B:	
Literature Describing Asthma Management Programs in Managed Care Organizations	195
Appendix C:	
Literature Describing Congestive Heart Failure Management Programs in Managed Care Organizations	212
Appendix D:	
Literature Describing Cardiovascular Disease Management Programs in Managed Care Organizations	225
Appendix E:	
Literature Describing Arthritis Management Programs in Managed Care Organizations	240
7. Conclusions and Future Research Directions	**255**
Observations on Existing Research	255
Research Challenges for the Future	260
Index	265
About the Authors	285

Foreword

This book represents the most detailed and critical look at the management of chronically ill individuals in managed care. Because of the rapid aging of the U.S. population and the increased survival of the chronically ill, the numbers of chronically ill and older patients are escalating, and their high health care costs have become a major political issue. Various forms of managed care now dominate many American markets. This review is timely given the increased public scrutiny of administrative and clinical strategies employed by managed care organizations (MCOs) and the retreat of many of these organizations from Medicare.

Are venal bureaucrats at health maintenance organizations (HMOs) threatening the health of our sickest citizens, as some have proclaimed? Are cost-cutting measures and constraints on physician decision making injuring those most in need of medical care? The published evidence reviewed by the authors provides little support for the notion that HMOs are more dangerous to the health of the chronically ill than American medical care in general. But, as the authors point out, most studies have examined care in more traditional managed care structures such as group- or staff-model HMOs.

Managed care has changed dramatically over the past two decades in response to market forces. The limited physician choice afforded by group and staff HMOs constrained their growth, leading to the development of new managed care models that provide broader physician choice. These newer IPAs, networks, and preferred provider organizations (PPOs), although they share the labels *managed care* and *HMO* with the traditional group- and staff-model organizations, differ in significant ways from their predecessors. These differences may have important implications for the care of the chronically ill (Wagner, 1997). The authors of this book argue forcefully for research that examines the effects of specific organizational and financial features of MCOs on the health and satisfaction of chronically ill patients.

Traditional group- or staff-model HMOs are integrated delivery and insurance systems whose physicians relate only to that organization. In such organizations, efforts to micromanage physician decisions through financial incentives and preauthorization review have largely been eschewed. Some of these organizations have been leaders in the search for innovative ways to better meet the needs of their patients with diabetes, HIV-AIDS, asthma, and other major chronic illnesses. Much of this experience is captured in the book. These strategies capitalize on the ability of these organizations to change practice systems and influence their clinicians to improve chronic-illness care (Wagner, Austin, & Von Korff, 1996). The authors correctly point out the limitations in the articles describing these innovations and the paucity of rigorously tested programs. Furthermore, many of the articles describe pilot efforts, with scant evidence that these innovations have had systemwide positive effects on patients. However, more recent studies have used more rigorous research designs, and evidence of systemwide impacts is beginning to appear in the literature (Brown, Nichols, & Glauber, 2000; McCulloch, Price, Hindmarsh, & Wagner, 2000; Petitti et al., 2000; Sperrl-Hillen et al., 2000).

IPAs and other managed care structures that involve large numbers of community physicians share only a few characteristics with traditional HMOs. IPA network and PPO physicians relate to multiple MCOs and, in many places, maintain sizable fee-for-service practices. Whereas joining a managed care medical group or staff has been and remains a significant career and cultural choice for a physician, joining a network or PPO is principally a financial transaction based on the market share and contract terms of the MCO. Because a given MCO insures only a small portion of the practice's clientele, care-management approaches attempt to directly influence or limit physician decision making for individual patients through financial incentives, utilization management, or referral of patients to disease-management companies. Conversely, the literature suggests that successful chronic-disease interventions generally require fundamental practice-system change involving alterations to the practice team and appointment and follow-up systems and the implementation of clear guidelines and disease registries (Wagner et al., 1996). In a practice contracting with multiple MCOs, a single health plan is very unlikely to influence the design of practice or, for that matter, clinical behavior. It is not surprising, then, that such organizations have not tended to be major sources of innovation and research in chronic-disease care. Research assessing the impacts of financial incentives, utilization review, disease-management carve-outs, and other MCO management strategies on patients with chronic illness is urgently needed.

Despite the limited number of high-quality studies, the authors point out the common features found in successful chronic-disease interventions. These correspond to the findings from other examinations of the chronic disease-management literature (Renders et al., 2001; Wagner et al., 1996) and include

1. Computerized data that enable measurement, care planning, reminders, and feedback that are essential underpinnings to population-based programs
2. Multidisciplinary teams with increased roles for nurses and pharmacists
3. Patient self-management support and involvement in the care process
4. Implementation of care guidelines

The book makes an important addition to the growing literature advocating more comprehensive system change to improve the outcomes of patients with chronic illness.

Although the book is the most complete and certainly the most critical review of the published literature on managed care of chronic disease, its scope and perspective should be considered by the reader. Other than comparative studies of fee-for-service versus HMO care, the research on "nonmanaged" chronic-illness care is not reviewed. The authors' criticisms of the methods and compass of research on managed care and chronic illness are well justified; however, the focus on managed care may lead some readers to believe that research on fee-for-service treatment of chronic disease is more rigorous and comprehensive. Such is not the case. In a study of best practices in the care of the chronically ill, for example, our group elicited nominations from a group of experts for the most innovative and effective chronic-disease programs in the United States (Wagner, Davis, Schaefer, Von Korff, & Austin, 1999). We studied 72 nominated programs, and fully one half were based in MCOs. Usually, the organization was a traditional HMO such as Kaiser Permanente or Harvard Pilgrim Health Care.

The contribution of traditional group or staff HMOs to progress in chronic-disease management may not be fully appreciated because of their shrinking role in marketplace. Regardless of the future of nonprofit group or staff HMOs, it may be wise to consider the organizational features of such organizations that have fostered innovations in chronic-illness care (Wagner, 1997). Such organizations have control over practices, dedicated clinicians, physician-led clinical cultures, centralized resources such as health education departments, and sophisticated data systems that facilitate system change and programmatic approaches to improving chronic-illness care. Some have invested in internal research organizations that incubate system improvements and have the research capacity to study them rigorously. It is these characteristics, in my view, that lead to chronic-disease improvement. This will be a hard row to hoe for IPA, network, and PPO models of managed health care, should they prevail.

Edward Wagner, M.D., M.P.H.
W. A. MacColl Institute for Health Care Innovation
Seattle, Washington

References

Brown, J. B., Nichols, G. A., & Glauber, H. S. (2000). Case-control study of 10 years of comprehensive diabetes care. *Western Journal of Medicine, 172*(2), 85-90.

McCulloch, D. K., Price, M. J., Hindmarsh, M., & Wagner, E. H. (2000). Improvement in diabetes care using an integrated population-based approach in a primary care setting. *Disease Management, 3,* 75-82.

Petitti, D. B., Contreras, R., Ziel, F. H., Dudl, J., Domurat, E. S., & Hyatt, J. A. Evaluation of the effect of performance monitoring and feedback on care process, utilization, and outcome. *Diabetes Care, 23*(2), 192-196.

Renders, C. M., Valk, G. D., Griffin, S. J., Wagner, E. H., van Eijk, J.T.M., & Assendelft, W.J.J. (2001). The effectiveness of interventions directed at improvement of the management of diabetes mellitus in primary care, outpatient, and community settings. In *Cochrane collaboration* (Issue 1). Oxford, UK: Cochrane Library.

Sperrl-Hillen, J., O'Connor, P. J., Carlson, R. R., Lawson, T. B., Halstenson, C., Crowson, T., & Wuorenma, J. (2000). Improving diabetes care in a large health care system: An enhanced primary care approach. *Joint Commission Journal on Quality Improvement, 26*(11), 615-622.

Wagner, E. H. (1997). Managed care and chronic illness: Health services research needs. *Health Serv Res, 32*(5), 702-714.

Wagner, E. H., Austin, A., & Von Korff, M. (1996). Organizing care for patients with chronic illness. *Milbank Quarterly, 74*(4), 1-34.

Wagner, E. H., Davis, C., Schaefer, J., Von Korff, M., & Austin, B. (1999). A survey of leading chronic disease management programs: Are they consistent with the literature? *Managed Care Quarterly, 7*(3), 56-66.

Preface

There has been a great deal of conjecture in the popular press and academic publications about the appropriateness of managed care as a philosophy, an organizing framework, and an operational approach for treating people with chronic illnesses. It is often hard to make sense of this discussion because what is encompassed by the term *managed care* typically is not clear. The discussion is frequently carried out without reference to empirical evidence on either side of the argument. Or, when study findings are referenced, it is difficult to determine how much faith to place in them. Was the study setting appropriate for the question? Was the study sample selected appropriately? Were the appropriate outcomes measured? Did the authors draw reasonable conclusions from their data? Are the results likely to be generalizable?

The purpose of this book is to help policy analysts, researchers, and practitioners better understand what is known, and not known, about a variety of topics relating to managed care and people with chronic illness. The structure of the book is described in detail in the first chapter. Like any critical literature review, however, the book has limitations that are important to note. First, it is constrained primarily to pieces published in the peer-reviewed literature, with a few important exceptions. This means that some studies that may be of interest to the reader are not included, and for that we apologize. Second, as with any literature review, there needs to be a cutoff point. We are aware of several important studies that were published after this manuscript was complete. Unfortunately, this will always be the case in a critical review of the type we have attempted here. Finally, in our review, we may not have been critical enough for some of our readers but may have been too critical for others. Again, this is a largely unavoidable problem, but one that we readily acknowledge. We hope that we have not misconstrued any of the studies we reviewed. In some cases, descriptions of study designs were quite limited, which frustrated our attempts to provide a critical assessment for our readers. If we misrepresented the studies we reviewed in any way, it was not intentional, and we apologize to the authors.

This book could not have been completed without the encouragement of many friends and colleagues at the Park Nicollet Institute. However, we want to especially recognize the unflagging support provided for our efforts by Jinnet Briggs Fowles, PhD, vice president, research, and James V. Toscano, executive vice president and chief operating officer. Without their support, this book would not have been undertaken, much less completed.

1 Introduction

The purpose of this book is to critically examine and summarize what is known, and not known, about how individuals with chronic illness are treated under managed care and about the outcomes of that treatment. The need for a critical examination of the research in this area seems clear. Chronic illness is recognized as a major health problem in the United States. Furthermore, the prevalence of chronic illness in the U.S. population is expected to increase with the aging of the "baby boomers" and the continued growth in life expectancy. Paralleling these trends is the growth in managed care and in the number of individuals who receive care through managed care organizations (MCOs), in the United States.

In a relatively short period of time, MCOs have become the dominant organizational structure for health care delivery in America. The approaches to care management pioneered by traditional health maintenance organizations (HMOs) have been adopted in other types of MCOs, and rapid developments in information technology have facilitated the use of a new generation of system-based approaches to care management as well (Gilbert, 1998; Svensk, 1996).

The rapid growth in managed care, and the replacement of traditional insurance options in employer benefits plans with MCOs, has contributed to a widely publicized managed care backlash. Physicians and patient advocacy groups have led the way in arguing that the management of care in MCOs is often ill-advised and overly aggressive, inappropriately usurping physician decision-making responsibilities and restricting patient choices. The American Medical Association (AMA) has suggested that physician unions may be necessary to represent physician and patient interests in negotiations with MCOs, while Congress is following the lead of many state legislatures in considering various versions of a patient "bill of rights."

Many of the issues being raised in the current debate about the promise and pitfalls of managed care echo concerns expressed 15 years ago about the advisability of treating individuals with chronic illnesses in MCOs. At that time, policy analysts noted that people with chronic illnesses are often in regular, frequent contact with the health care system and typically are more expensive to care for than average enrollees in MCOs. The careful management of their treatment could potentially save dollars for MCOs while at the same time improving the health status of patients. However, inappropriate restrictions on treatment could have immediate deleterious effects on these patients, because of their need to access a broad array of health care resources and their relatively precarious health status. Furthermore, according to these analysts, people with chronic conditions might be unable or unwilling to advocate for themselves aggressively in interactions with an MCO over benefit coverage or treatment regimen. Or, MCOs might seek to avoid enrolling chronically ill people in the belief that they cost more to care for than the "average" enrollee.

For these reasons, it is important to understand how MCOs care for people with chronic illness and the effects of that care on health status. In this book, we report the findings of a critical review and synthesis of the existing literature on this subject. This is a challenging task in several respects, not the least of which is the shifting, somewhat ambiguous use of the terms *chronic illness* and *managed care*. We begin by discussing these concepts and the definitions we relied on to guide us in our review. Then, in the remainder of the chapter, we describe the process we used to search for relevant research studies and to organize the results of that search.

Defining Chronic Illness

Definitions of chronic illness and, by extension, chronic illness treatment often emphasize what chronic illness is not; that is, they focus on how chronic illness is different from acute illness. An acute illness is a condition that can be cured, with the potential of returning the patient to normal functioning within a relatively short period of time. Medical care is organized and directed toward achieving this result. In the broadest view, chronic illness is any condition that does not fit this description. More narrowly, it is a condition that is expected to persist, with medical care directed at symptom control or delay of further deterioration in patient health.

This broad definition of chronic illness has been used quite commonly, either implicitly or explicitly, by health care analysts. In an oft-cited study of the costs associated with chronic illness, health services researchers Hoffman, Rice, and Sung (1996) identify individuals in the National Medical Expenditure Survey (1987) with chronic illness by noting the presence of some physical or mental impairment or a diagnosis code "that is not self-limiting, but creates persistent and recurring health consequences, lasting for periods of years (not days or months)" (p. 474).

In an analysis of ethical issues involved in treating patients with chronic illnesses, Jennings, Callahan, and Caplan (1988) define a chronic illness as

> a condition that lasts for a substantial period of time. It is also commonly defined as a condition that interferes with daily functioning for more than three months a year, causes hospitalization for thirty days or more per year, or (at the time of diagnosis) is likely to do either of these. (p. 4)

They observe that this definition encompasses a wide variety of different illnesses with different causes, symptoms, and effects on patient lifestyle.

Charged with guiding the Health Care Financing Administration (HCFA) in policy decisions regarding health plans and their treatment of patients with complicated illness, the Institute of Medicine of the National Academy of Sciences defined a "serious and complex condition" as "one that is persistent, substantially disabling or life threatening, and that requires treatments and interventions across a broad scope of medical, social and mental health services" (Chrvala & Sharfstein, 1999, p. 2). Note that "serious and complex" conditions could encompass acute problems not usually classified as chronic in the literature.

Peter Conrad (1987), in reviewing the sociological literature on chronic illness, observes that "some sociologists have attempted to bypass medical definitions and develop sociologically meaningful categories of study" (p. 23). Sociology's focus is on the social and psychological aspects of living with chronic illness, leading Conrad to distinguish between "lived with" illnesses and other chronic illnesses. The former refers to an illness that "a person must adapt to and learn to live with but which is (usually) not life-threatening" (p. 24). It excludes what Conrad terms *mortal illnesses,* which are life threatening (e.g., cancer), and *at-risk illnesses* such as hypertension.

Finally, for the study of the epidemiology of chronic illnesses, other definitional approaches have been employed. For example, Rothenberg and Koplan (1990) argue, "No axiomatic definition exists for chronic diseases, but these diseases are well described by their attributes: long latency, protracted clinical course, uncertain etiology and no definitive 'cure'." (p. 267). However, the authors note that "the clinical notion of chronicity is reflected in the epidemologic characteristics of most chronic diseases: gradual changes in secular trends, asynchronous evolution, and heterogeneity in population susceptibility" (p. 267).

In focusing our literature review and synthesis, we confine ourselves primarily to "lived with" illnesses. Specifically, we focus on five major conditions: diabetes, asthma, congestive heart failure (CHF), arthritis (osteo and rheumatoid), and cardiovascular disease (including hypertension, dyslipidemia, and coronary artery disease [CAD]). The illnesses we address contribute to a substantial amount of overall health care spending in the United States, and therefore their management is likely to receive the attention of MCOs. For instance, diabetes alone has been estimated to account for about 15% of U.S. health care expenditures (Quickel, 1996). We do not include mortal illnesses, although the dividing line between mortal and "lived with" is not always clear. For instance, we include CHF in our review because patients with CHF can survive over a period of years if the illness is managed properly. However, there is also a reasonably high risk of death from this condition. We also include hypertension (even though Conrad would exclude it) because it is commonly termed a chronic illness in the medical literature.

Largely for practical reasons, we exclude two types of illnesses that sometimes are classified as chronic. Their inclusion would expand the scope of this review substantially. These include illnesses that are chronic but relatively rare and all types of mental illnesses. The latter, along with substance abuse, will be addressed in a separate book in this series.

Defining Managed Care/ Managed Care Organizations

Just as there appears to be no general consensus on the definition of chronic illness, the term *managed care* has been used in the literature to represent various concepts. This reflects, in part, an evolving public familiarity with MCOs, but it also is symptomatic of the ongoing development of new managed care techniques and new organizational structures and relationships within which these techniques are applied.

During the 1970s, the HMO was the prototype MCO, although the terms *managed care* and *managed care organization* were largely absent from the literature. Luft (1981) described an HMO as an organization that integrated the functions of insurance and health care provision, and this basic notion has persisted in many current definitions of managed care. Individuals who enrolled in an HMO entered into a contract with an administrative entity for the delivery of medical services by a circumscribed network of providers for a fixed fee. Great attention was given to the fact that HMOs were prepaid and thus were at financial risk for costs associated with excessive use of medical services. HMOs organized around salaried physicians (e.g., Group Health of Puget Sound) or a single physician group in a geographic area (e.g., Kaiser Health Plans in the various Kaiser regions); they were expected to manage care in a way that kept costs below prepaid amounts and yet resulted in acceptable levels of quality.

This early depiction of an HMO, where there was little attempt to distinguish between organization (e.g., MCO) and method of health care delivery (e.g., managed care), has carried over to some recent definitions of managed care as well. For instance, in an educational document prepared for health policy makers, the National Council of State Legislatures says that managed care is "a term that describes health care systems that integrate the financing and delivery of appropriate health care services to covered individuals by arrangements with selected providers" (Harden, 1994, p. 2) and then continues with a listing of activities often engaged in by these systems. Also during the early 1990s, a "Glossary of Terms" published by a large, for-profit health care corporation defines managed care as "a system of health care delivery that influences utilization of services, cost of services, and measures of performance" (United Health Care Corporation, 1992, p. 41). While both of these definitions explicitly equate managed care with health care systems, neither focuses on a specific payment mechanism as essential to the concept. This suggests that, over time, the general notion of managed care has evolved to encompass a broad set of activities not tied to capitation or a specific organizational form such as an HMO.

Further evolution is reflected in two recent definitions. In *The Managed Health Care Dictionary,* Richard Rognehaugh (1998) defines managed care as

> any method of health care delivery designed to reduce unnecessary utilization of services and provide for cost containment while ensuring that high quality care or performance is maintained; a system to minimize cost of care and "churning" while still delivering good access to high quality health care. (p. 134)

The first part of Rognehaugh's definition emphasizes that managed care constitutes a method of health care delivery, rather than an organization. This approach is underscored by Peter Fox (1997), in Kongstvedt's well-known textbook, *Essentials of Managed Health Care.* Fox states that

> When one thinks of managed care, one should distinguish between the techniques of managed care and the organization that performs the various functions. Managed care can embody a wide variety of techniques . . . these include various forms of financial incentives for

providers, promotion of wellness, early identification of disease, patient education, self-care, and all aspects of utilization management. A wide variety of organizations can implement managed care techniques [and] a variety of hybrid arrangements have evolved [that are difficult to characterize]. (pp. 3-4)

The movement away from thinking about managed care as imbedded in certain types of health care organizations (e.g., HMOs) or health care delivery systems seems particularly appropriate, given the changing nature of what are commonly thought of as MCOs. In discussing "The Future of the Managed Care Organization," Robinson (1999) observes that "systems incorporating both insurance and delivery are to be found more frequently in health policy proposals than in the managed care marketplace" (p. 18). The insurance function is often assumed by employers (particularly larger employers) in contracts with MCOs, whereas MCO contracts with providers often shift utilization management responsibilities to the provider organization. Some research suggests that these provider organizations employ the same utilization management techniques as traditional MCOs, when faced with the challenge of providing care under risk contracts (Kerr et al., 1995). As Robinson (1999) puts it, "Health maintenance organizations (HMOs) and other insurers are hollowing out, yielding one function after another to purchasers and providers" (p. 8). When this occurs, firms traditionally thought of as MCOs may do little to actually *manage* care.

In our review, where possible, we will use the term managed care in the sense advocated by Fox; that is, as a set of techniques used to influence the delivery of health services to a defined population. However, we also are constrained by the study designs in the articles we review, as well as the common meaning of the term managed care during the time period in which the study was conducted. For instance, during the 1980s, studies of the impact of managed care on people with chronic illness typically compared HMO enrollees to fee-for-service insurance beneficiaries. In many of these studies, managed care was simply "whatever HMOs did." In contrast, several recent studies have focused on the patient outcomes associated with applying a particular utilization or demand management approach within a provider organization. These studies provide important information about the relationship between managed care and chronic illnesses. We include studies of this type in our review when they are identified through our search process.

Organizing the Literature Review and Synthesis

The literature review begins in Chapter 2 with a synthesis of articles written by health care analysts, policy makers, patient and managed care advocates, and medical care providers that identify potential strengths and issues related to managed care and the treatment of patients with chronic illnesses. These articles address, on the one hand, concerns about the ability of MCOs to deliver appropriate care to people with chronic illnesses and, on the other hand, the potential for MCOs to improve on the care such patients receive. The chapter attempts to present these often conflicting views in an organized and unbiased way. This discussion is used to identify topics that guide the literature reviews in the chapters that follow.

Chapter 3 focuses primarily on research that compares the performance of MCOs in treating people with chronic illness to that of fee-for-service medicine. In most cases, this research was carried out when MCOs served a relatively small proportion of the population and the HMO was the dominant form of MCO. In this research literature, comparisons are carried out at the system or organizational level and contrast cost, process, and outcomes of care. Typically, these studies are not designed to assess what specific approaches or strategies used by MCOs are effective, or problematic, in treating people with chronic illness. Although early studies of this type compare patients in a single HMO to fee-for-service patients, more recent studies use data from multiple MCOs and compare patients by MCO type as well as MCO versus fee-for-service. This shift reflects the increasing dominance of MCOs in the health insurance market, along with the development and popularity of MCO alternatives to the HMO.

In Chapter 4, we document what is known about the prevalence in MCOs of different chronic illness management techniques and programs. Based largely on the self-reports of MCOs, these studies provide an overview of MCOs' strategies designed to improve chronic illness treatment. But, they are limited in the detail they contain regarding specific structures or initiatives and their effectiveness.

In Chapter 5, we shift emphasis to what is known about the different approaches used within MCOs to deliver care to enrollees with chronic illnesses. As a first step, we review the literature that compares the performance of a specific MCO in caring for its chronically ill members to either an explicit benchmark or to past performance. These studies typically rely on administrative data sets (claims) maintained by the MCO for payment purposes and often, they are conducted by research groups within MCOs. In essence, most attempt to describe "usual care" for people with chronic illness within a particular MCO.

Chapter 6 moves the analysis down to the microlevel, focusing on interventions or programs implemented in managed care settings. There is a growing literature that consists of evaluations of specific chronic illness treatment programs implemented in a variety of environments. Early studies of this type tended to be carried out in academic medical centers or large urban hospitals. More recently, however, an increasing number of studies have been conducted within MCOs, or within physician organizations, hospital systems, or integrated delivery systems that contract with MCOs on a risk basis to serve an enrolled population. The number of such studies varies considerably across type of chronic illness, with diabetes and asthma receiving the most attention. Our review of this literature summarizes what is known about the effectiveness of these chronic illness management initiatives.

The final chapter in the book goes beyond the review and critique of published research. It underscores the difficulties researchers face in conducting rigorous evaluations of MCO initiatives to manage chronic illnesses and formulates research questions relating to the treatment of chronic illnesses in MCOs. The focus is on identifying questions that have received limited attention, or have not been addressed at all, in published studies to date. The chapter highlights for policy makers topics on which more information is needed in an attempt to stimulate new research in these areas. The chapter describes changes in the environment and in the structures of MCOs that are now occurring, or are likely to occur in the near future, and briefly discusses the opportunities these changes could create for new research.

Searching for Relevant Literature

To identify literature reviewed for this volume, we conducted targeted searches of the Medline® and HealthStar databases. The Medline® database, published by the U.S. National Library of Medicine, includes information from three print indexes: Index Medicus, Index to Dental Literature, and International Nursing Index. In addition, Medline® also includes bibliographic references from the biologic and physical sciences, humanities, and information sciences as they relate to health and medicine. HealthStar is published jointly by the National Library of Medicine (NLM) and the American Hospital Association. In addition to the resources encompassed by Medline®, HealthStar provides access to nonclinical sources of information regarding health care financing, planning, and administration.

The literature review includes primarily studies published in the past 15 years, although publications produced prior to this date were included if they are considered to be landmark studies or "classics" in the field. A final update of the literature review was conducted in March 2000 to identify additional publications catalogued in the NLM databases that were published in 1999.

The literature we reviewed consists primarily of publications from peer-reviewed, academic journals. For the overview of MCO disease management initiatives (Chapter 4) and the review of specific disease management interventions (Chapter 6), however, some publications from non-peer reviewed journals were included. Innovative disease management programs not otherwise described in peer-reviewed studies, or in non-peer reviewed reports of disease management initiatives where rigorous research methodologies were employed, were sometimes included to provide a more complete picture of disease management activities as they are occurring currently throughout the United States.

Literature for Chapters 2 through 5 was gathered using keyword searches of the following terms in various combinations: managed care (and derivatives: prospective payment system, managed care programs, HMO, Health Maintenance Organization, group practice, prepaid health plans), chronic illness/disease management, health status, health outcomes, outcomes assessment (health care), Medical Outcomes Study (MOS), Medicare Demonstration, Medicare competition, delivery of healthcare, economic competition, consumer participation, capitation fee, and surveys. Each of these terms (or combination of terms) was cross-referenced with searches for five individual disease categories of interest (diabetes, asthma, CHF, arthritis, cardiovascular disease) and any pertinent terms specific to these conditions (insulin-dependent diabetes mellitus [IDDM], non-insulin dependent diabetes mellitus [NIDDM], osteoarthritis, rheumatoid arthritis, lipids, hyperlipidemia, dyslipidemia, hypertension, CAD, anticoagulation).

Chapter 6 presents a review of disease management programs specifically related to the management of CHF, cardiovascular disease, diabetes mellitus, asthma, and arthritis. (See the appendix to this chapter for a brief description of each of these illnesses.) Literature for Chapter 6 was identified using search terms to identify these diseases, in combination with the following key words: managed care (and all derivatives: prospective payment system, managed care programs, HMO, Health Maintenance Organization, group practice, prepaid health plans), disease management, team management, and management. Interventions included in this review are restricted to those implemented in the United States.

APPENDIX:
Description of Illnesses

Diabetes

Diabetes mellitus results from the pancreas not producing enough insulin or the body not properly using insulin that is produced from the pancreas. The pancreas is a gland that lies behind the stomach. Insulin is a hormone made by the pancreas that helps the body use glucose for energy. The hallmark of diabetes mellitus is an elevated blood sugar. There are two type of diabetes:

Type I diabetes. Often referred to as insulin dependent diabetes mellitus (IDDM), Type I diabetes used to be called early onset or juvenile-onset diabetes. Type I diabetes occurs when the pancreas makes little or no insulin. People with Type I diabetes must have insulin injections every day. Although this illness is more common in children or young adults, anyone can have Type I diabetes. Type I diabetics represent about 10% of the diabetic population.

Type 2 diabetes. About 90% of all diabetics have Type 2 diabetes, formerly known as adult-onset diabetes. Type 2 diabetes occurs when the body does not properly use the insulin that the pancreas manufactures. Type 2 diabetes may at times be controlled with diet or with oral medications rather than insulin injections. Although Type 2 diabetes is often referred to as non-insulin dependent diabetes mellitus (NIDDM), this is a misnomer, as many Type 2 diabetics must use insulin to control their blood sugar.

The long-term complications of diabetes include blindness (because of diabetic retinopathy), heart disease, nephropathy, neuropathy, and limb amputations. In the short term, diabetics are vulnerable to non-healing wounds and various infections. Both the long-term and short-term complications of diabetes, however, can be greatly mitigated by proper control of blood-sugar levels (The Diabetes Control and Complications Trial Research Group, 1993; Lasker, 1993; Mazze, Bergenstal, & Ginsberg, 1995; McCulloch, Glasgow, Hampson, & Wagner, 1994).

The successful control of diabetes requires intensive self-management by patients in the form of home blood-glucose self-monitoring and, particularly in the case of Type 1 diabetics, self-adjustment of medications. Diabetic patients must also manage their condition with careful diet and exercise. Intensive self-management by patients must be coupled with extensive patient education and vigilant monitoring by health care providers (Etzwiler, 1972; Mazzuca et al., 1986; Rosenstock, 1985). The glycosylated hemoglobin test (referred to in this book as the HbA1c) provides a 12- to 14-week view of blood-glucose control. Nondiabetics generally have an HbA1c ranging from 4% to 6%. HbA1c levels below 8% are generally considered to represent good control in diabetic patients (although levels of 6% are vastly more desirable than levels of 8%). The 8% to 10% range is generally considered moderate to poor control, and levels above 10% are considered very poor control.

In addition to regular HbA1c testing (four times per year for Type 1 diabetics and at least two times per year for Type 2 diabetics), the American Diabetes Association recommends a series of regular evaluations for diabetic patients including annual foot examinations, ophthalmic examinations, and lipid testing. Unfortunately, as reported in Chapter 6, these tests are conducted in fewer than 60% of diabetic patients in many care settings (both managed care and non-managed care) (Chicoye, Roethel, Hatch, & Wesolowski, 1998; Rubin, Dietrich, & Hawk, 1998).

Although the onset of Type 1 diabetes is quickly detected, an individual may have Type 2 diabetes for several years without knowing it. It has been estimated that those adults who have been officially diagnosed with Type 2 diabetes represent only 50% of all adults who actually have the condition.

Cardiovascular Disease (CVD)

Cardiovascular disease (CVD) refers to a constellation of conditions involving the heart and surrounding vessels. Among the most prevalent of these is coronary artery disease (CAD). CAD occurs when the arteries of the heart, the coronary arteries, contain blockages. CAD may cause angina or chest pain with exertion. CAD may also cause a heart attack or CHF. Cholesterol and blood clots that collect inside the arteries cause CAD. When the arteries become narrow or blocked, they cannot transmit oxygen to the heart muscle, and part of the heart muscle is damaged or dies. CAD is more common in men older than 50 and in postmenopausal women. Risk factors for CAD include smoking, diabetes, elevated LDL cholesterol, low HDL cholesterol, or a family history of early CAD.

Regular aspirin use is often recommended for CAD patients, and beta blockers are viewed as the first-line therapy for patients with stable disease. Where beta blockers are contraindicated, patients are often prescribed long-acting nitrates. Patient education is an important key to the management of CAD. Patients need education regarding the course of the disease and need to be trained to recognize worsening symptoms. Patients must be instructed in the use of aspirin and nitroglycerin where appropriate. Patients must also be encouraged to stop smoking, to maintain an ideal body weight, and to sustain appropriate activity levels.

Asthma

Reversible narrowing of the air passages in the lungs causes asthma. Pollen, dust, animal dander, molds, some foods, respiratory infections, and exposure to smoke, exercise, or emotional stress may trigger asthma. Repeat attacks are common, with inflammation of the airways causing the narrowing. Asthma may be associated with other allergic problems, such as eczema and hay fever. The symptoms of asthma include wheezing, shortness of breath, and cough. At times, asthma may be life threatening.

Asthma is best diagnosed through spirometry in patients 5 years and older. In terms of severity, asthma is diagnosed as mild intermittent, mild persistent, moderate persistent, or severe persistent.

The most recommended strategy for managing mild to severe asthma involves the regular use of inhaled corticosteriods supplemented by inhaled beta agonists for acute attacks (Lozano & Lieu, 1999; Sullivan et al., 1996). Severe asthmatics may include long-acting bronchiodilators in this regimen. Often, particularly among child asthmatics, medications are not administered correctly. Proper education about the use of medications and the use of spacer devices and metered dose inhalers (MDIs) can help ensure proper delivery of medications. Many asthma care specialists also advocate the use of peak-flow monitoring by patients at home (Homer, 1997; Lozano & Lieu, 1999; O'Brien, 1997; Self & Nolan, 1997). Another useful management strategy, particularly for children, involves the development of a written action plan, which patients (and their parents) can use as a guide when asthma symptoms set in (Plaut, Howell, Walsh, Pastor, & Jones, 1996).

The most common complicating factor in the management of asthma arises from the failure of patients to take their maintenance medications for the prevention of attacks. Rather, many patients wait for the onset of an acute attack to treat their asthma. It is important to note that many asthmatics do not know that they have asthma until the onset of a severe attack. The frequency of early recognition and diagnosis of asthma varies greatly by race and ethnicity in the United States.

Arthritis

Arthritis refers to inflammation of joints. Osteoarthritis, which affects nearly 16 million Americans, and rheumatoid arthritis are the two most prevalent forms of arthritis (Bilodeau, 1995; Hirano, Laurent, & Lorig, 1994). Arthritis causes painful and swollen joints and at times may permanently damage joints. Among those over 65, 49% of Americans are estimated to have arthritis, according to the National Health Interview Survey (Bilodeau, 1995).

Osteoarthritis is also called degenerative joint disease or "wear and tear" arthritis. Cartilage that usually cushions the joint becomes soft and breaks down. This may lead to redness, swelling, and pain in the joints. The cause of this disease is not known, but it is very common in people older than age 50. The joints typically involved in arthritis include knees, hips, wrists, and knuckles.

Rheumatoid arthritis results from the immune system attacking the lining of joints. Compared to osteoarthritis, it more frequently involves small joints. At times, rheumatoid arthritis can lead to progressive joint damage.

Monitoring of medication use and patient education are the primary methods of managing both rheumatoid and osteoarthritis. Medication side effects can be severe in some patients, and recently developed medications for arthritis management offer new hope to patients who could not tolerate the older pharmaceutical agents. Patient education as a disease management strategy for arthritis has been investigated in-depth. Primarily, other types of disease management strategies for arthritis have not been widely developed because there is little evidence regarding the effectiveness of arthritis treatments on which to base disease management efforts.

Patient education interventions appear to increase patients' knowledge and self-efficacy, improve health behaviors, and decrease perceived pain; however, the connection between patient education for arthritis management and actual improvements in health status or management of arthritis remains largely undemonstrated (Hawley, 1995; Hirano et al., 1994). But because arthritis is a progressive condition, it could be argued that educational interventions for the disease cannot be expected to improve objective measures of health status. Rather, improvements in patient self-efficacy, behavior, and perceived pain may be suitable end goals for arthritis management.

Congestive Heart Failure (CHF)

CHF occurs when the heart does not function adequately as a pump. As the pumping action of the heart weakens, fluid may build up in the lungs and in the legs. In addition, the brain and muscles may not receive an adequate blood supply when the pumping action of the heart weakens. Symptoms of CHF include shortness of breath with exertion, sudden shortness of breath at night, swelling of the legs, and muscle fatigue. Common causes of CHF include damage to the heart from longstanding high blood pressure or from heart attack.

It is estimated that 5 million Americans, or 1.9% of the total population, have been diagnosed with CHF, and 400,000 new cases are diagnosed each year (National Heart, Lung, and Blood Institute, 1996; Wilkes, Dukes, Feagles, Leong, & Allen, 1999). CHF is the primary cause in 43,000 deaths each year and is a contributing cause in an additional 220,000 deaths each year (National Heart, Lung, and Blood Institute, 1996). The cost of treating CHF in the United States has been estimated to range between $10 billion and $40 billion annually (Abraham & Bristow, 1997; American Heart Association, 1998).

CHF is a particularly pervasive problem among those older than age 65 and is the leading discharge diagnosis for hospitalized individuals in this age group (Abraham & Bristow, 1997; Wilkes et al., 1999).

There exists a widely recognized set of evidence-based guidelines for CHF management, particularly in the area of pharmacotherapy. ACE inhibitors are universally recommended as the first line of therapy for CHF patients with both systolic and diastolic dysfunction in all functional classes, including asymptomatic patients. Hydralazine Isosorbide Dinitrate is recommended for patients with systolic dysfunction who are intolerant of ACE inhibitors. Second only to ACE inhibitor therapy is the recognized importance of diuretic use in patients with both systolic and diastolic dysfunction. Other evidence-based pharmacological management guidelines include Digoxin for patients with atrial fibrillation, third heart sound, or left ventricular dilation and beta-blockers for patients whose symptoms persist after the use of ACE inhibitors.

The evidence for nonpharmacological therapies for CHF treatment is not as strong as that for pharmacotherapies, although recommendations exist. A sodium-restricted diet, sometimes with fluid restriction, is recommended for most patients. It is also recommended that patients pursue a moderate exercise program (after adequate screening), reduce stress, and monitor daily weight gain.

Patient education regarding symptom recognition and medication management is also an important component of CHF management.

Despite the existence of a well-established set of guidelines for CHF management, evidence suggests that compliance among practitioners with these guidelines is low. Patient compliance with recommended regimens is also frequently poor.

References

Abraham, W. T., & Bristow, M. R. (1997). Specialized centers for heart failure management [Editorial]. *Circulation, 96*(9), 2755-2757.
American Heart Association. (1998). *Heart and stroke statistical update, 1998*. Dallas, TX: Author.
Bilodeau, A. (1995). Easing the pain of arthritis. *HMO, 36*(4), 70-74.
Chicoye, L., Roethel, C. R., Hatch, M. H., & Wesolowski, W. (1998). Diabetes care management: A managed care approach. *WMJ, 97*(3), 32-34.
Chrvala, C. A., & Sharfstein, S. (Eds.). (1999). *Definition of serious and complex medical conditions*. Washington, DC: National Academy Press.
Conrad, P. (1987). The experience of illness: Recent and new directions. *Research in the Sociology of Health Care, 196*, 1-31.
The Diabetes Control and Complications Trial Research Group. (1993). The effect of intensive treatment of diabetes on the development and progression of long-term complications in insulin-dependent diabetes mellitus. *New England Journal of Medicine, 329*(14), 977-986.
Etzwiler, D. D. (1972). The patient is a member of the medical team. *Journal of the American Dietetic Association, 61*(4), 421-423.
Fox, P. (1997). An overview of managed care. In P. Kongstvedt (Ed.), *Essentials of managed care*. Gaithersburg, MD: Aspen.
Gilbert, J. A. (1998). Disease management hits home. *Health Data Management, 6*(8), 54-60.
Harden, S. (1994). *What legislators need to know about managed care*. Denver, CO: National Council of State Legislatures.
Hawley, D. J. (1995). Psycho-educational interventions in the treatment of arthritis. *Baillieres Clinical Rheumatology, 9*(4), 803-823.

Hirano, P. C., Laurent, D. D., & Lorig, K. (1994). Arthritis patient education studies, 1987-1991: A review of the literature. *Patient Education and Counseling, 24*(1), 9-54.

Hoffman, C., Rice, D., & Sung, H. Y. (1996). Persons with chronic conditions: Their prevalence and costs. *Journal of the American Medical Association, 276*(18), 1473-1479.

Homer, C. J. (1997). Asthma disease management. *New England Journal of Medicine, 337*(20), 1461-1463.

Jennings, B., Callahan, D., & Caplan, A. L. (1988). Ethical challenges of chronic illness. *Hastings Center Report, 18*(1/suppl), 16.

Kerr, E., Mittman, B., Hays, R., Siu, A., Leake, B., & Brook, R. (1995). Managed care and capitation in California: How do physicians at financial risk control their own utilization? *Annals of Internal Medicine, 123*(7), 500-504.

Lasker, R. D. (1993). The diabetes control and complications trial: Implications for policy and practice. *New England Journal of Medicine, 329*(14), 1035-1036.

Lozano, P., & Lieu, T. A. (1999). Asthma in managed care. *Pediatric Annals, 28*(1), 74-80.

Luft, H. (1981). *Health maintenance organizations: Dimensions of performance*. New York: John Wiley.

Mazze, R. S., Bergenstal, R., & Ginsberg, B. (1995). Intensified diabetes management: Lessons from the diabetes control and complications trial. *International Journal of Clinical Pharmacology and Therapeutics, 33*(1), 43-51.

Mazzuca, S. A., Moorman, N. H., Wheeler, M. L., Norton, J. A., Fineberg, N. S., Vinicor, F., Cohen, S. J., & Clark, C. M., Jr. (1986). The diabetes education study: A controlled trial of the effects of diabetes patient education. *Diabetes Care, 9*(1), 1-10.

McCulloch, D. K., Glasgow, R. E., Hampson, S. E., & Wagner, E. (1994). A systematic approach to diabetes management in the post-DCCT era. *Diabetes Care, 17*(7), 765-769.

National Heart, Lung, and Blood Institute. (1996). *Congestive heart failure in the United States: A new epidemic*. Bethesda, MD: U.S. Department of Health and Human Services.

O'Brien, K. P. (1997). Asthma in the managed care setting. *Current Opinion in Pulmonary Medicine, 3*(1), 56-60.

Plaut, T. F., Howell, T., Walsh, S., Pastor, M., & Jones, T. (1996). A systems approach to asthma care. *Managed Care Quarterly, 4*(3), 6-18.

Quickel, K. E., Jr. (1996). Managed care and diabetes, with special attention to the issue of who should provide care. *Transactions of the American Clinical and Climatology Association, 108* 184-195.

Robinson, J. (1999). The future of the managed care organization. *Health Affairs, 18*(2), 7-24.

Rognehaugh, R. (1998). *The managed health care dictionary* (2nd ed.). Gaithersburg, MD: Aspen.

Rosenstock, I. M. (1985). Understanding and enhancing patient compliance with diabetic regimens. *Diabetes Care, 8*(6), 610-616.

Rothenberg, R. B., & Koplan, J. P. (1990). Chronic disease in the 1990s. *Annual Review of Public Health, 11,* 267-296.

Rubin, R. J., Dietrich, K. A., & Hawk, A. D. (1998). Clinical and economic impact of implementing a comprehensive diabetes management program in managed care. *Journal of Clinical Endocrinology and Metabolism, 83*(8), 2635-2642.

Self, T., & Nolan, S. (1997). Long-term management of asthma: How to improve outcomes. *American Journal of Managed Care, 3*(9), 1425-1438.

Sullivan, S., Elixhauser, A., Buist, A. S., Luce, B. R., Eisenberg, J., & Weiss, K. B. (1996). National Asthma Education and Prevention Program working group report on the cost-effectiveness of asthma care. *American Journal of Respiratory and Critical Care Medicine, 154*(3, Part 2), S84-S95.

Svensk, U. (1996). Disease management at the system level—an effective way to improve health care. *International Journal of Health Care Quality Assurance, 9*(7), 4-8.

United Health Care Corporation. (1992). *A glossary of terms: The language of managed care and organized health care systems.* Minnetonka, MN: Author.

Wilkes, R. M, Dukes, K. R., Feagles, L. L., Leong, D., & Allen, G. L. (1999). Kaiser Permanente's approach to congestive heart failure in south San Francisco. *Journal of Clinical Outcomes Management, 6*(5), 37-40.

2 Chronic Illness and Managed Care: What Are the Issues?

In the first chapter, we noted that two parallel trends underscore the importance of critically examining the treatment, under managed care, of people with chronic illness: the recent and projected growth in the number of people with chronic illnesses in the United States and in the number of people receiving their medical services under some form of managed care. In this chapter, we discuss these two trends in greater detail, to provide a context for the concerns that have been raised by policy analysts, physicians, and others. These concerns relate to the potential impact on chronically ill patients, and the care they receive, of the financial incentives and utilization management approaches associated with managed care. We then use this summary as an organizing framework for our assessment of the findings in the empirical literature, as presented in the chapters that follow.

People With Chronic Illness

Using a definition of chronic illness that is broader than the one we use in this book, Hoffman, Rice, and Sung (1996) concluded that, in 1987, people with impairments or conditions that are not self-limiting constituted 46% of the noninstitutionalized population in the United States. One third of young adults, two thirds of the middle-aged population, and 88% of the 65-and-older population had at least one chronic condition. Even more important as it relates to the potential use of health services, 44% of people with chronic conditions had more than one, with 69% of the elderly having more than one. As one might expect, the value of the resources used in treating people with chronic conditions is considerable. In their work, Hoffman et al. (1996) estimate that total annual expenditures for medical services and supplies were about $272 billion in 1987 dollars, with private insurance covering about one third of this cost. Other policy analysts have attempted to estimate costs specific to the treatment of some common chronic illnesses. For instance, Quickel (1996) cites literature suggesting that expenditures for diabetic people in the United States in 1992 were $105 billion, with direct costs for medical treatment totaling $45 billion.

As impressive as these dollar amounts are, they are expected to increase significantly over the next 10 to 30 years, with the aging of the population. Life expectancy at birth increased from 69.7 years in 1960 to 75.5 years in 1993, with the number of elderly growing from 16.6 million to 32.8 million (Hoffman et al., 1996). People 65 years and older are now about 13% of the U.S. population, and this will increase to 20% by 2030 as the postwar baby boom cohort ages (Allen, Fennell, & Laliberte, 1998). As noted above, the elderly are more likely to have chronic conditions and to have more than one condition. In addition to projected increases in the demand for care that will accompany the aging of the population, care demands may increase due to an increasing prevalence of some chronic illnesses within certain population subgroups.

The growing demands for treatment of chronic illnesses would likely strain the U.S. medical care system, with or without managed care. This is because, as Kane (1999) observes, "medical care in this country has been operating as if we were still in an era of acute care when the reality clearly indicates that we entered an era of chronic disease long ago" (p. 35). Wagner, Austin, and Von Korff (1996) note that medical practices are typically organized to respond to acute needs, with a reliance on patient-initiated visits and an emphasis on symptom relief. Physicians lack adequate training in the treatment of people with chronic illnesses, and the financial rewards physicians receive typically are not commensurate with the rewards for treating patients with acute illnesses. The result is that care too often is fragmented and episodic, with an overuse of expensive diagnostic and therapeutic strategies and an underemphasis on patient education and involvement in the care process (Sandy & Gibson, 1996). In commenting on this situation, Vinicor (1998) asserts that there is a substantial gap between what is known to be efficacious treatment for asthma and diabetes mellitus and the daily practice of care, suggesting that mortality and morbidity could be reduced if what is known were put into practice. Overlaying these concerns about the ability of the medical care system to respond appropriately to increasing numbers of people with chronic illness is the rapid shift in the structure and orientation of that system toward managed care.

The Shift to Managed Care

In the private sector, the shift of enrollment of individuals into health insurance options and accompanying delivery systems that embody, to some degree, features associated with managed care has been startling in its pace. From 1987 to 1997, the percentage of the employed population in purely fee-for-service, unmanaged insurance plans dropped from 95% to 18%, with a corresponding increase in the percentage in some form of managed care arrangement (Brenden & Hamer, 1998). Included in these managed care organizations (MCOs) are tightly structured staff-model health maintenance organizations (HMOs) (now few in number), more loosely organized independent physician association (IPA)-model HMOs, Preferred Provider Organizations (PPOs), and so-called managed indemnity plans. The latter are insurance arrangements that pay providers on a fee-for-service basis, offer access to a broad range of providers, but attempt to employ various utilization management techniques to control costs. HMO enrollment alone grew from 25.8 million in 1987 to 78.8 million in 1998 (InterStudy, 1999), whereas the number of HMOs grew from 265 in 1987 to 651 in 1997 (Brenden & Hamer, 1998). Data on enrollment in other types of MCOs are less readily available, but an annual survey conducted by the SMG consulting group provides some indication of PPO popularity (Hoechst Marion Roussel, 1998). In 1997, there were 1,035 PPOs in the United States, an increase of 5% from 1996. About 60% were owned by insurance companies. PPOs provided health insurance coverage to about 89 million people in 1997.

A number of interesting aspects to this growth in managed care bear on the concerns that we summarize in the sections to follow. First, although MCOs typically were included in employee health-benefits offerings as an alternative to relatively unmanaged health insurance options in the past, this often is no longer the case. A substantial portion of small employers, in particular, now offer their employees only a single MCO (Jensen, Morrisey, Gaffrey, & Liston, 1997). This means that larger numbers of people with chronic illnesses can no longer opt out of managed care arrangements when choosing insurance coverage. Second, until recently, the use of capitation to pay primary-care physicians in HMOs was on the rise, as was the requirement that primary-care physicians act as gatekeepers. Under capitation, an individual physician or a provider group receives a fixed payment per time period to serve designated enrollees in the HMO, rather than being paid each time a service is provided. Typically, under the gatekeeper approach, the patient enrolls with a primary-care physician on entry into the HMO and must seek a referral from that physician to see a specialist (Gold, Hurley, Lake, Ensor, & Berenson, 1995; InterStudy, 1999). More recently, however, the cost-effectiveness of gatekeeping has been called into question by some large MCOs that are adopting an "open access" approach to specialty care. Also, some MCOs appear to be modifying their gatekeeper policies in response to consumer dissatisfaction.

Third, although early HMOs featured minimal patient cost sharing in the form of deductibles or co-payments, this is not true of newer forms of MCOs, such as PPOs and managed indemnity plans (Gabel, 1997). Much of the recent growth in enrollment in managed care plans has been in these newer forms, which also feature broader provider networks and looser controls on utilization.

Fourth, over the past 10 years, the HMO industry has been transformed from predominantly nonprofit to predominantly for-profit. At the same time, enrollment has shifted from locally based entities to national firms (InterStudy, 1999). There also has been an increase in the number of specialized MCOs that serve individuals with specific types of illnesses, including some that focus on specific chronic illnesses (see Chapter 5).

Fifth, the use of practice guidelines and other evidence-based tools to influence utilization has increased, as has the emphasis on information systems to support physician practices. Indeed, these efforts are now viewed by some as the hallmark of managed care and as more effective than financial incentives in influencing physician behavior (Wagner, 1996).

Finally, and perhaps most important, managed care is becoming much more prevalent in public health insurance programs for the elderly (Medicare) and the poor (Medicaid). As noted earlier, older people are more likely to have chronic conditions and to have more than one chronic condition.

MCOs receive a fixed payment per month from Medicare to enroll beneficiaries and may charge enrollees a premium as well. Beyond a minimum set of required benefits, MCOs may choose to offer additional coverage to attract enrollees. Coverage of prescription drugs, which is of particular interest to beneficiaries with chronic illness, is currently a discretionary benefit that may or may not be covered under the enrollee's premium payment. Currently, MCOs do not receive a higher payment from Medicare when they enroll chronically ill beneficiaries.

Contracts between Medicaid programs and MCOs have increased in number over the past 5 years (InterStudy, 1999). From the perspective of state Medicaid programs, these fixed payment contracts make Medicaid program expenditures more predictable and hold the potential for reducing upward trends in expenditures. As with Medicare, there are subgroups of Medicaid beneficiaries with a high incidence of chronic illness, and payment from Medicaid typically is not higher for MCOs enrolling these beneficiaries. The subgroup that has received the most attention consists of children with asthma. Unlike Medicare, MCOs may not charge beneficiaries a premium for supplemental Medicaid payments. Managing care for beneficiaries with chronic illness is complicated by the substantial amount of movement on and off of Medicaid eligibility. This is a particular issue in the treatment of chronic illnesses, where continuity of care is thought to be desirable.

Early Concerns

Early commentators on how people with chronic illnesses would fare under managed care relied primarily on theoretical arguments relating to the potential impact of managed care payment incentives and utilization-control mechanisms on treatment processes and, ultimately, patient outcomes. This approach was reasonable, given the early stages of development in the managed care industry and the relatively small number of studies that documented how MCOs treated chronically ill individuals. It also reflected the prevailing perception of managed care, where the integration of financing and delivery was seen as the differentiating feature of MCOs, and these organizations were seen as alternatives to the traditional system of indemnity insurance, which featured unrestricted access to providers. There was substantial agreement (in these discussions) that the traditional system could be improved, as it related to the treatment of people with chronic illnesses. Several limitations were noted, including fragmentation in the delivery of care, with little or no incentive for providers to coordinate service delivery; often substantial co-payments and deductibles in insurance policies, which discouraged chronically ill people from seeking care; lack of patient education and involvement in their own care; and inadequate training of physicians in diagnosing and treating chronic illnesses. With this as a framework, arguments were advanced concerning whether chronically ill patients treated under managed care (or, more accurately, enrolled in MCOs) were likely to fare better or worse than similar patients in the existing system. The conclusion of these assessments was, typically, that there was cause for concern and that chronically ill patients were particularly vulnerable to under-service in MCOs, if they were able to enroll in these organizations at all.

Potential for Improvement Over Usual Care

The potential of MCOs to improve the treatment of people with chronic illness, as early commentaries portrayed it, was primarily due to the fact that these organizations were paid on a capitation basis and structured to facilitate collaboration among physicians in patient care. Under capitation, MCOs receive a per-person, per-month payment to provide all necessary medical care through their employed or contracted providers. In theory, this creates an incentive for MCOs to see that care is coordinated, as coordinated care presumably would be less expensive than the fragmented care that characterized the traditional system (Fox & Fama, 1996). Coordination of care, as epitomized in a "care team" approach, was seen as particularly beneficial for people with chronic illnesses or multiple illnesses, because they often require treatment from multiple providers of different types in different locations (Schlesinger, 1986). Capitation also provides an incentive for MCOs to employ a variety of treatment resources to meet the needs of chronically ill patients. Under the traditional system, health insurance policies covered primarily medical services. In theory, MCOs receiving capitation payments could choose to pay for social or rehabilitative services if these services were deemed appropriate for the patient (Sandy & Gibson, 1996). Thus, in MCOs, the range of treatment resources available to chronically ill patients could expand. Finally, HMOs at that time did not require deductibles or co-payments from their members, with the exception of small amounts per visit or per filled prescription. Therefore, chronically ill people enrolled in HMOs did not face financial barriers that discouraged them from seeking care in a timely manner.

Another feature of managed care that argued for potential improvement over usual care was the structure of the delivery systems within many MCOs. In the 1970s, and through the early 1980s, the larger, better known MCOs were staff- or group-model HMOs. In these organizations, physicians practiced as part of a multispecialty group and were reimbursed on a salaried basis. In theory, this practice environment reinforced the potential benefits flowing from capitation payment as they related to the treatment of chronically ill people. Arguably, it would be easier to coordinate care among physicians practicing in the same group, and often in the same location, than among solo practice physicians in different locations. Furthermore, there were no financial incentives for individual physicians to retain patients when a referral would be more appropriate, and there were opportunities for informal as well as formal consultations over treatment plans (Wagner, 1996).

In summary, although enrolling chronically ill people in group- or staff-model HMOs under capitation-payment arrangements would not address all of the perceived shortcomings of their treatment under the existing system (e.g., inadequate physician training in the treatment of chronic conditions), it clearly offered the potential for improvement. However, most commentators also saw substantial impediments to achieving this potential and, in fact, a considerable risk that chronically ill people would fare worse under managed care.

Potential Limitations and Shortcomings of Managed Care

Early skeptics regarding the ability of managed care to improve the treatment of people with chronic illness emphasized three points: MCOs were not available to portions of the population where the prevalence of some chronic illnesses was high; where they were available, MCOs would try to avoid enrolling people with chronic illnesses; and MCOs would unduly restrict access to services for people with chronic illness who did enroll. With respect to the first point, during the 1980s, there were relatively few MCOs that served Medicare or Medicaid beneficiaries. Chronic illnesses such as congestive heart failure (CHF) and diabetes are especially prevalent in the aged population, and asthma is especially prevalent among low-income children. Because MCOs were rarely available to Medicaid and Medicare beneficiaries, the potential positive impact of managed care on people with chronic illnesses was limited, assuming that, on balance, its impact was positive. Those who argued that managed care's impact was likely to be negative would view its relative absence from public programs as desirable.

The second and more controversial point was the suggestion that MCOs would be able to avoid enrolling, to some degree, people with chronic illnesses in the employed population, including dependents (Fox & Fama, 1996). This argument is a variation on the general idea that MCOs can increase their profits if they can avoid enrolling "bad risks" and instead enroll a disproportionate share of "good risks" in an employed group, with chronically ill people decidedly in the bad-risk category. In most employed settings, there is an annual open-enrollment period during which employees select their health insurance arrangement for the coming year (assuming the employer offers more than one arrangement). In the 1980s, large employers typically offered their employees a choice of one or more managed care options in conjunction with a traditional insurance plan. A managed care plan could not deny enrollment to an employee who selected it during an open-enrollment period. However, it was argued that MCOs could encourage the enrollment of relatively healthy employees and dependents and discourage the enrollment of sicker employees, including those with chronic illnesses, through their marketing approaches and the way in which they structured their provider networks and care management processes. For example, if MCOs excluded from their provider networks physician groups that were well-known for their treatment of specific chronic illnesses (e.g., diabetes), this could make MCOs less attractive to enrollees with those illnesses. From a financial standpoint, MCOs might view this as desirable because, compared to other potential enrollees, people with chronic illnesses are relatively costly (Caldwell, 1993). Given that MCOs have a fixed amount of dollars to spend on their enrolled populations, attracting a disproportionate share of chronically ill people could threaten their financial viability, if it resulted in higher-than-budgeted medical care costs. In markets where there are multiple competing MCOs, raising premiums in subsequent periods to recoup losses may not be possible. Therefore, according to this line of reasoning, MCOs have financial incentives to avoid enrolling people with chronic illnesses, to the degree that this is possible, and to encourage the disenrollment of those who do join their plans.

For the same reason that MCOs may wish to avoid enrolling people with chronic illnesses, some commentators have argued that MCOs may inappropriately limit services for those who do enroll (Schlesinger, 1986; Schlesinger & Mechanic, 1993). According to this argument, the potential advantages of MCOs in the treatment of chronic illnesses are likely to evaporate under pressures to contain costs. For instance, rather than acting as coordinators of care for chronically ill patients, primary-care physicians frequently are called on to function as gatekeepers. That is, the policies of the MCO may require chronically ill patients to see their primary-care physician for a referral before visiting a specialist (Barr, 1995; Caldwell, 1993; Schlesinger & Mechanic, 1993). This gives the primary-care physician the opportunity to "close the gate" on access to specialty care for the treatment of chronic illness. Similarly, in an effort to control costs, MCOs may deny reimbursement for nonmedical services, limiting, rather than expanding, the range of services available to people with chronic illnesses (Schlesinger, 1986; Schlesinger &

Mechanic, 1993). In this scenario, care for chronically ill people will remain relatively uncoordinated within MCOs, access to care will become more difficult, and more chronically ill people will go without needed care.

Current Debate

The current debate has evolved considerably from early commentaries, reflecting in part the changing nature of MCOs and managed care processes and in part the accumulation of experience on the part of providers and others with the treatment of chronically ill people under managed care. Although serious concerns are still expressed about the potential effect of managed-care payment arrangements on access to and use of services, there is also an acknowledgement that the processes used by some MCOs to manage the care of enrolled populations could benefit people with chronic illnesses (Quickel, 1996). However, there is skepticism regarding whether these processes can or will be employed effectively for these populations, given the incentives facing some MCOs and the current structure of the managed care industry.

Potential for Improvement Over Usual Care

From a positive perspective, early commentators emphasized the potential for capitated payments to group- or staff-model HMOs to improve the integration and coordination of care and extend the range of services available to people with chronic illnesses. More recently, the emphasis has shifted to the potential for MCOs to lead the effort to strengthen and disseminate evidence-based approaches for the treatment of chronically ill people (Jacobs, 1998). There is accumulating research evidence that various types of treatment interventions can be successful in improving the health status of chronically ill people and their overall satisfaction with their lives and the care they receive. MCOs, using quality-improvement processes supported by sophisticated information systems, in theory can facilitate the development and dissemination of treatment guidelines and identify substandard treatment processes or inappropriate medication use. By adopting a systems approach to care management, they arguably can identify, within their defined population of enrollees, people who have specific chronic illnesses and allocate resources appropriately to manage their care. Writing regarding hypertension management, Jacobs (1998) summarizes this viewpoint:

> Managed care provides opportunities for coordinated care grounded in evidence-based medicine rather than in ad hoc, anecdote-based decisions . . . [I]n managed care systems, an increasing emphasis on both patient and physician accountability is replacing the patient and physician autonomy inherent in the old system. (pp. S749-S750)

Referring to diabetes management by HMOs, Quickel (1996) observes that "because HMOs have more control over physician practice patterns, tend to have more sophisticated data support systems, and often use the necessary ancillary staff, they have the potential for better diabetes care if they choose to provide it" (p. 162).

The development of private-sector efforts to evaluate MCO performance systematically along a variety of dimensions, including chronic illness treatment, and to reward MCOs that do well, is viewed by some as a positive development in creating systems accountability for the management of chronic illness. Many employers are now demanding accreditation by the National Committee on Quality Assurance (NCQA) before they will offer MCOs as health benefit options for their employees (Sennett, 1998). MCOs receive points toward accreditation if they meet population-based performance standards, some of which relate to the treatment of people with chronic illnesses. For instance, in the Health Plan Employer Data and Information Set (HEDIS) version 3.0, there are two measures of quality related to the treatment of chronic conditions of the type reviewed in this book (hospitalization rates for childhood asthma and annual eye examinations for diabetics). The risk inherent in this process is that MCOs may devote disproportionate resources to improving NCQA measures for specific chronic illnesses, shifting resources away from the treatment of other chronic illnesses where performance is more difficult to assess (Wagner et al., 1996).

Potential Limitations and Shortcomings of Managed Care

Current critics of MCOs conclude that they will not fulfill their potential in the management of chronic illness, in large part because they continue to focus on cost minimization and profits to the detriment of chronically ill members. Critics see recent changes in the managed care marketplace as supporting this conclusion. For instance, Clough (1997) asserts that

> In its current incarnation, managed care has a major flaw: it fails to address the health care needs of people with chronic disease, for whom prevention is too late. So far, the current system of managed care, with its focus on minimalist care and short-term outcomes and its prejudice against using expensive specialists, has failed to address this unfortunate segment of the population, except to erect new and often obnoxious hurdles to block their access to necessary care. (p. 67)

Others point out that treatment interventions demonstrated to improve the health status of chronically ill people have diffused very slowly into standard practice. In part, they attribute this to the ascendancy, in the current marketplace, of IPA-model HMOs and PPOs. One reason that these types of MCOs are favored by consumers is that they generally offer access to a large network of providers. People with chronic illnesses are more likely to find their primary-care physician or their specialist of choice in an IPA or PPO network than in a network offered by a group- or staff-model HMO. However, increased within-network choice has potential drawbacks for these patients. Physicians in IPAs/PPOs maintain their own independent, geographically separate practices and typically contract with multiple MCOs. This makes the implementation of targeted intervention programs and clinical guidelines designed to improve chronic illness care more difficult than under staff- or group-model HMOs; physician commitment to the programs and guidelines of any single MCO is not likely to be strong.

It is also true that IPAs/PPOs often are part of for-profit, national managed care companies. Some commentators have expressed concern that the focus of these companies on short-term gains for shareholders discourages investment in programs to improve treatment for people with chronic illnesses. In a pragmatic sense, MCOs may find it difficult to make a business case for investing in new treatment programs and supportive infrastructure (Shulkin, 1999), in part because the financial benefits from these efforts, driven by the avoidance of future service use, may be speculative and, in any case, will take some time to be realized (Jacobs, 1998). Also, the standard accounting processes used in MCOs may not readily capture these possible financial benefits. Even where a strong case can be made for the existence of a future financial return on the investment in treatment programs, that return may not be captured by the investing MCO, due to enrollee switching among MCOs. This may explain Kane's conclusion that "unfortunately, managed care has turned out to be an insurance reform, not a clinical one. Clinically, it is still business as usual, but with more attention to the short-term bottom line" (p. 37).

In addition to these issues, in the present managed care environment, capitation-payment arrangements between purchasers and MCOs of all types, and their potential effect on people with chronic illnesses, remain a concern. MCOs continue to have incentives for avoiding enrollees with chronic illnesses, who predictably would consume large amounts of resources, unless their payments can be adjusted to reflect these additional costs. Hillman (1995) observes that "risk-adjustment entails predicting the cost to be incurred by certain populations in a statistically reliable fashion and adjusting capitation rates (and other budgets) to reflect this level of resource use" (p. S27). Several approaches to risk adjustment are currently under way, some of which focus on adjusting payments for people with chronic conditions (e.g., see Kronick, Zhou, & Dreyfus, 1995, for a discussion of risk-adjusted payments for Medicaid beneficiaries with chronic illnesses). Successful risk adjustment would weaken incentives for MCOs to avoid enrollees with chronic illness, but skeptics observe that this is not happening at present and question the likelihood that it can be implemented in the near future (Schlesinger & Mechanic, 1993).

Even under risk-adjusted payment, capitated MCOs are at risk for spending in excess of the capitated amount and are rewarded, in the short run, for delivering fewer services. A minority of IPA-model HMOs have attempted to manage their financial risk by shifting a significant portion of it to primary-care physicians. These physicians receive capitated payments for each enrollee designating the physician as his or her primary-care provider. In effect, this pushes the incentives implicit in capitation payment down from the MCO or the medical group level to the individual physician. If the capitation payment includes allowances for laboratory tests or specialist services, the primary-care physician receives a relatively direct financial reward for restricting the use of services. This is regarded as a particularly problematic set of financial incentives when treating people with chronic illnesses, because these patients often require regular laboratory tests and access to specialists (Schlesinger & Mechanic, 1993). Although these concerns are real, recent data suggest that capitation arrangements of this type are not common and may be declining in popularity. Where they do exist, their impact is typically softened by various types of reinsurance and stop-loss arrangements that limit individual physician losses associated with high-cost patients.

The potentially negative impact of capitation arrangements on treatment of people with chronic illness may be diminishing in importance. So-called open-access plans appear to be gaining in popularity, at least in the insured employed population. Under these plans, physicians are typically paid on a fee-for-service basis, and enrollees can access specialists directly (e.g., Wood, 1999). Open-access plans reduce concerns about physician payment incentives that could restrict access to specialists for people with chronic illnesses, but they raise other issues. In particular, effective coordination of care between primary-care physicians and specialists may be harder to achieve in open-access plans.

The elimination of choice of MCOs for some employees is a feature of the evolving managed care industry that also could be detrimental to people with chronic illnesses. If these people are forced to switch into an MCO from a managed indemnity plan, or move from an MCO with a broad panel to one with a more constrained choice of providers, in theory, they could lose access to their physician of choice and have the continuity of their care disrupted. In practice, employers offering only one health plan option—an MCO—frequently offer an IPA with a large physician network, or a point-of-service HMO product, or a PPO. Under the latter two options, chronically ill patients can retain their physicians but may have to pay more for each visit or procedure if the physician is not in the MCO network. Additional costs also could be incurred in obtaining medications, if the new MCO has a more restrictive formulary. These additional costs could discourage access to needed services or medications or result in a shift to a less preferred provider, from the patient's perspective.

Finally, a recent market development has been the emergence of managed care companies that specialize in treating individual chronic illnesses, with diabetes being the most common (Blumenthal & Buntin, 1998; Cave, 1995). MCOs or large employers may choose to carve out their enrollees with a given chronic illness and contract, under a capitated-payment arrangement, with a firm that specializes in the treatment of people with that illness. One presumed benefit to patients of this arrangement is that the providers employed by the firm are experts in the treatment of their illness. Also, the firm can provide a continuum of treatment services and has special expertise in medication management and in monitoring and evaluating patient progress. Apparently, very few of these carve-out arrangements exist in practice at this time (Blumenthal & Buntin, 1998). Nevertheless, some analysts suggest that, because these firms typically focus on treating a single chronic illness and it is common for chronically ill patients to have multiple problems, coordination of care is likely to suffer (HMO Workgroup, 1998), and fragmentation of care could result. Fragmentation of care is also seen as a potential problem in MCOs that employ "carve in" programs to treat patients with chronic illness. The concern is that these highly targeted internal programs could result in treatment of the patient's chronic illness separately from the overall medical management of the patient.

Research Issues

The ongoing debate in the literature regarding the potential impact of managed care on the treatment of people with chronic illnesses and their resulting health outcomes raises a variety of issues that could be clarified through research. These issues are summarized in Table 2.1. In the chapters that follow, we review the existing literature to determine

Table 2.1 Research Questions Suggested by the Literature

Early Period

1. Is care for people with chronic illnesses coordinated more effectively, or less effectively, in managed care organizations (MCOs) than under traditional insurance arrangements?
2. Is there a broader or narrower range of treatment resources, medical and nonmedical, used by patients with chronic illnesses in MCOs versus those who have traditional insurance arrangements?
3. Are more or fewer medical (and nonmedical) services sought and received by people with chronic illnesses in MCOs versus those who have traditional insurance arrangements?
4. Where MCOs are available, are people with chronic illnesses enrolled in higher or lower proportions than they are present in relevant population subgroups?
5. Are patients with chronic illnesses who are enrolled in MCOs more or less likely to be treated by specialists than if they were covered by traditional insurance arrangements? Are referrals to specialists more or less likely to be appropriate when the patient is an MCO enrollee?
6. How does health status for people with chronic illness enrolled in MCOs compare to the status of similar people who have traditional insurance arrangements? Does enrollment in an MCO have a positive or negative impact on the health status of people with chronic illnesses?

Current Debate

1. To what degree are MCOs using systems approaches to identify people with chronic illnesses and support their treatment? Where these approaches have been used, is there evidence that they yield improvements in patient outcomes or reductions in costs compared to usual care?
2. What is the evidence that MCOs attempt to manage care for chronically ill members using promising treatment models? Have chronically ill people benefited from participation in these programs? Have resources been saved? Does this vary by type of MCO, type of chronic illness, or presence of multiple conditions?
3. How prevalent are managed care companies that treat patients with specific chronic illnesses? What is the evidence of their effectiveness?

the degree to which these issues are addressed and to identify other issues that may have been posed by researchers. Where a research literature exists relating to a specific issue, we assess the breadth of that literature along with the strengths and limitations of the individual studies that we think are the most significant. Our objective is to reach conclusions, based on research findings, concerning what is known, and not known, about a given issue. We also comment about the likely appropriateness of generalizing from those findings to different treatment settings, populations, or types of managed care or MCOs.

References

Allen, S. M., Fennell, M., & Laliberte, L. (1998). The impact of managed care on chronic care agency providers. *Medicine and Health, Rhode Island, 81*(3), 87-90.

Barr, D. A. (1995). The effects of organizational structure on primary care outcomes under managed care. *Annals of Internal Medicine, 122*(5), 353-359.

Blumenthal, D., & Buntin, M. B. (1998). Carve outs: Definition, experience, and choice among candidate conditions. *American Journal of Managed Care, 4*(Suppl), SP45-57.

Brenden, J., & Hamer, R. (1998, August). The InterStudy HMO trend report: 1987-1997. Bloomington, MN: InterStudy Publications.

Caldwell, J. R. (1993). Who is to serve? The chronically ill patient in the managed care milieu [Editorial]. *The Journal of the Florida Medical Association, 80*(8), 523-524.

Cave, D. G. (1995). Capitated chronic disease management programs: A new market for pharmaceutical companies. *Benefits Quarterly, 11*(3), 6-23.

Clough, J. D. (1997). Chronic disease management and managed care: Specialists have an important role [Editorial]. *Cleveland Clinic Journal of Medicine, 64*(2), 67-68.

Fox, P. D., & Fama, T. (1996). Managed care and chronic illness: An overview. *Managed Care Quarterly, 4*(2), 1-4.

Gabel, J. (1997, May/June). Ten ways HMOs have changed during the 1990s. *Health Affairs, 16*(1), 134-145.

Gold, M. R., Hurley, R., Lake, T., Ensor, T., & Berenson, R. (1995, December 21). A national survey of the arrangements managed care plans make with physicians. *New England Journal of Medicine, 353*(25), 1678-1683.

Hillman, A. L. (1995). The impact of physician financial incentives on high-risk populations in managed care. *Journal of Acquired Immune Deficiency Syndromes and Human Retrovirology, 8*(Suppl 1), 523-530.

HMO Workgroup on Care Management. (1998, March). Essential components of geriatric care provided through health maintenance organizations. *Journal of the American Geriatrics Society, 46*(3), 303-308.

Hoechst Marion Roussel. (1998). *Managed Care Digest Series™ 1998: HMO-PPO/Medicare-Medicaid digest.* Kansas City, MO: Author.

Hoffman, C., Rice, D., & Sung, H. Y. (1996). Persons with chronic conditions: Their prevalence and costs. *Journal of the American Medical Association, 276*(18), 1473-1479.

InterStudy. (1999, April). *The InterStudy competitive edge, Part II: HMO industry report.* Bloomington, MN: Author.

Jacobs, R. (1998, December). Hypertension and managed care. *The American Journal of Managed Care, 4*(12) (supplement), 749-756.

Jensen, G., Morrisey, M., Gaffrey, S., & Liston, D. (1997, January/February). The new dominance of managed care: Insurance trends in the 1990s. *Health Affairs, 16*(1), 125-130.

Kane, R. (1999, Summer). A new model of chronic care. *Generations, 23*(2), 35-37.
Kronick R., Zhou Z., & Dreyfus T. (1995, Spring). Making risk adjustment work for everyone. *Inquiry, 32*(1), 41-55.
Quickel, K. E., Jr. (1996). Diabetes in a managed care system. *Annals of Internal Medicine, 124*(1, Part 2), 160-163.
Sandy, L. G., & Gibson, R. (1996). Managed care and chronic care: Challenges and opportunities. *Managed Care Quarterly, 4*(2) 5-11.
Schlesinger, M. (1986). On the limits of expanding health care reform: Chronic care in prepaid settings. *Milbank Quarterly, 64*(2), 189-215.
Schlesinger, M., & Mechanic, D. (1993). Challenges for managed competition from chronic illness. *Health Affairs (Project Hope), 12*(Suppl), 123-137.
Sennett, C. (1998). Measuring health plans' performance in chronic care (Interview). *The Quality Letter for Healthcare Leaders, 10*(9), 10-12.
Shulkin, D. J. (1999). Understanding the economics of succeeding in disease management. *Managed Care Interface, 12*(4), 98-104.
Vinicor, F. (1998). Diabetes mellitus and asthma: "Twin" challenges for public health and managed care systems. *American Journal of Preventive Medicine, 14*(3) (Suppl), 87-92.
Wagner, E. H. (1996). The promise and performance of HMOs in improving outcomes in older adults. *Journal of the American Geriatric Society, 44*(10), 1251-1257.
Wagner, E. H., Austin, B. T., & Von Korff, M. (1996). Organizing care for patients with chronic illness. *Milbank Quarterly, 74*(4), 511-544.
Wood, K. (1999, January/February). Blue Shield of California's Access One HMO. *Health Affairs, 18*(1), 174-177.

3 Individuals With Chronic Illness

MCO Versus Fee-for-Service Comparisons

From the 1970s through the 1980s, and even into the early 1990s, as more Americans enrolled in managed care organizations (MCOs) and MCO models proliferated, research attention naturally focused on whether people with chronic illness were being enrolled in these new systems, how they were being treated, and whether their health was being affected. The approach taken in most studies that addressed any of these questions was to compare a group of individuals with a particular chronic illness or combination of illnesses who were enrolled in MCOs to a similar group not enrolled in MCOs. Until the mid-1980s, this research focused primarily on comparisons of enrollees in a single health maintenance organization (HMO) (sometimes called prepaid care) with individuals in the same geographic area being treated under traditional insurance arrangements (sometimes called indemnity insurance or fee for service). After the mid-1980s, as enrollment in new types of HMOs expanded and new MCO models such as PPOs became important organizational vehicles for delivering managed care, this approach was modified to a degree. Some researchers expanded the scope of their study designs to include multiple HMOs operating in multiple markets and, in some instances, to compare outcomes of interest between different HMOs, different types of HMOs, and MCOs and traditional insurance. However, PPOs and other newer MCO models typically have not been evaluated in published, peer-reviewed studies.

Our review of this literature found studies that addressed several of the early-period research questions listed in Table 2.1.

- Where MCOs are available, do people with chronic illness choose to enroll in them?
- At any point in time, are people with chronic illnesses present in MCOs in higher or lower proportions than they are present in relevant comparison groups?
- Are more or fewer medical (and nonmedical) services sought and received by people with chronic illnesses in MCOs versus those covered by traditional insurance arrangements?
- Are people enrolled in MCOs as likely to be treated by specialists for their illness as people with traditional insurance arrangements?
- How does health status for people with chronic illness enrolled in MCOs compare to the status of similar people in traditional insurance arrangements?
- Does enrollment in an MCO have a positive or negative impact on the health status of people with chronic illnesses?

We found no studies relating to two general issues that were identified as important in the early debate about managed care and chronic illness, as summarized in Chapter 2: coordination of care and availability of a range of treatment resources.

In this chapter, we discuss the published, peer-reviewed literature in the research areas noted above. In addition to describing these studies, their findings, and their strengths and weaknesses, we point out where there are significant areas of consensus and where there are substantial gaps in our knowledge.

Given a choice, do people with chronic illness enroll in MCOs? Are people with chronic illness present in MCOs in higher or lower proportions than they are present in relevant comparison groups?

The first question addresses the issue of whether, given a choice, people with chronic illness are more likely to select traditional insurance arrangements or MCOs. If they are more likely to select traditional insurance arrangements, this would suggest that MCOs benefit from favorable selection, assuming that people with chronic illness require more services and cost more than the "average" person in the enrollment pool. People with chronic illness who fear that MCOs may restrict their access to preferred medications and specialists might prefer traditional insurance arrangements over MCOs, leading to favorable selection for MCOs. On the other hand, MCOs typically require lower out-of-pocket payments for physician visits and pharmaceuticals, and this might be sufficiently attractive to people with chronic illnesses to overcome concerns about access limitations, resulting in adverse selection for MCOs. In other words, there are incentives for people with chronic illness to favor as well as to avoid MCOs when choosing a health plan.

A large number of studies have attempted to determine the factors that influence individuals in their choice of health plans. Some of these studies, in part due to the limitations of the statistical methodology they employ, focus their attention on the influence of health-plan characteristics on plan choice. Others include a range of consumer characteristics as variables that might possibly influence health-plan choices. A subset of these studies use measures of the health status of individuals as predictors of health-plan choice, with an even smaller number including indicators of the presence of chronic illness or different types of chronic illnesses. In 1986, Wilensky and Rossiter summarized the literature on health-plan choice as it relates to the question of favorable selection. They concluded that the early literature provided mixed evidence concerning whether HMOs attract healthier people. Later studies, however, indicated that HMOs did attract a disproportionate share of individuals with lower health risks from among enrollment groups. These authors discussed some of the limitations of employing prior service use or self-perceived health status as measures of health for the purposes of analyzing factors influencing health-plan choice, but they did not explicitly discuss the use of chronic illness measures in the studies they reviewed. The Wilensky and Rossiter review was updated and expanded by Hellinger in 1995. Hellinger not only considered studies of enrollment choice in HMOs but also reviewed the limited literature about enrollment in PPOs. He concluded that plans that restricted their provider networks received favorable selection because "individuals who consume large amounts of health resources often are unwilling to sever ties with their health care providers" (p. 135). Although there was no specific mention of people with chronic illness, it is reasonable to assume that they would be categorized as "individuals who consume large amounts of health resources," at least if measured over time.

Most of the major studies of health-plan choice do not directly control for the presence or absence of chronic conditions in individuals making the choice (Buchmueller & Feldstein, 1997; Davidson, Sofaer, & Gertler, 1992; Grazier, Richardson, Martin, & Diehr, 1986; Hennelly & Boxerman, 1983; Long, Settle, & Wrightson, 1988; McGuire, 1981; Scanlon, Chernew, & Lave, 1997; Short & Taylor, 1989; Welch & Frank, 1986). Three studies do introduce a measure of the presence of a chronic condition, and their findings are mixed. In the earliest of these studies, Juba, Lave, and Shaddy (1980) examined the decision of Carnegie Mellon University employees the first time they were offered the option of enrolling in an HMO (1976). They found that the number of family members reporting an illness requiring regular or repeated medication or medical treatment had a positive effect on the probability of choosing an HMO. However, in a finding they labeled "apparently inconsistent," they also concluded that lower self-reported health status reduced the probability of selecting an HMO.

Merrill, Jackson, and Reuter (1985) studied enrollment decisions of state employees in Tallahassee, Florida, and Salt Lake City, Utah. (The year in which the data were collected is not specified in the article.) In their Tallahassee sample, they found that the greater the number of different chronic conditions in a family, the more likely the family was to select the HMO, where the HMO had a relatively limited provider network. But, this relationship was not statistically significant in the Salt Lake City sample, where the HMO was an independent physician association (IPA) model with a broad provider network. In Tallahassee, prescription drug coverage was not offered in the HMO but was offered in the indemnity plan. However, there was more cost sharing in the Tallahassee indemnity plan than in the HMO option. These findings suggest that, in the early stages of development of the HMO industry, there were features of HMOs that were attractive to people with chronic illness, although the evidence is not strong. There is no information provided by the authors about the care management activities of the HMOs in their study but, given the time period, these were likely to have focused on inpatient care and may not have been viewed as especially pertinent to people with chronic illnesses, who required regular outpatient care.

In 1989, Feldman, Finch, Dowd, and Cassou (1989) studied the enrollment decisions of employees in 17 Minneapolis firms, using data collected in 1984. The HMO options available to these employees included IPAs and group- or staff-model plans. In their analysis, they included a control variable defined as presence of a "longstanding medical condition for which regular care or medicines are used." About 22% of their sample reported the presence of such a condition. In their analysis of family health-plan selection decisions, a condition was said to exist if anyone in the family reported one. They did not find any evidence that presence of a chronic condition, using their measures, affected choice of health plan.

In summary, the literature on whether people with chronic illnesses are more or less likely to join MCOs is equivocal. Studies that used general measures of health status found some evidence that less healthy people were less likely to select MCOs, when given an option. The most commonly used measures of health status were self-reports (e.g., excellent, good, fair, or poor health) or costs or service use in a prior period. However, people reporting poor health or using large amounts of services in a prior period may have experienced, or might be experiencing, an acute illness episode. Therefore, these measures are crude proxies, at best, for the presence of chronic illness. There have been relatively few attempts to control more directly for the presence of chronic illness in studies of health-plan enrollment decisions, and the measures that have been used in these studies also are somewhat crude. Nevertheless, the studies did not find evidence that individuals with chronic illnesses were less likely to select MCOs. The data used in these studies were pre-1990, however, and therefore may reflect an environment in which health plans were less aggressive in managing outpatient care than they were in subsequent years.

The second question addresses an issue closely related to that addressed by the first question. It asks whether, at any point in time, the proportion of enrollees in MCOs with chronic illnesses is similar to, or different from, that which can be observed in a comparison group. Sometimes, the comparison group is chosen to be representative of the general population within a selected age range. More typically, however, the comparison group consists of the subset of the general population that is not enrolled in MCOs or in a particular type of MCO. One would expect the general conclusions of these studies to be consistent with the results summarized above relating to the health-plan choice. That is, because there was no consistent evidence that people with chronic illness were more or less likely to select MCOs, it seems logical to expect that, at any point in time, they would be present among MCO enrollees and comparison groups in similar proportions. However, it is certainly possible that differences could exist. For instance, although people with chronic illnesses may be equally likely to enroll in MCOs and traditional insurance arrangements, once enrolled, they may differ in the rate in which they experience chronic illnesses over time or the rate at which they disenroll. This could lead to differences in proportions of enrollees with chronic illness at a point in time even though, at the time of enrollment, chronically ill people didn't sort into one type of insurance arrangement versus another.

A number of studies provide data on enrollees in single MCOs versus traditional insurance alternatives. They vary greatly in their sophistication, and many are severely limited in their generalizability. We have chosen to discuss only those studies that are relatively broad in scope, either due to the use of samples that cover large geographic areas and/or the use of data from multiple MCOs. An early study related to the second question was conducted by Dowd and Feldman (1985). They compared the proportion of enrollees in three types of health plans (traditional insurance arrangements, IPA model HMOs, and group- or staff-model HMOs) who had long-standing medical conditions such as hypertension, allergies, diabetes, or arthritis. Their data were collected from 5,161 employees in 20 non-randomly selected large employers in the Minneapolis/St. Paul area. Dowd and Feldman found that compared to MCOs, traditional insurance arrangements had a higher proportion of enrollees with chronic illness, under both single and family coverages. The prepaid group and IPA-model HMOs did not differ significantly in the presence of chronic illness among their enrollees.

An analysis of this type with a broader geographical base was published by Kravitz et al. (1992) as part of the Medical Outcomes Study. This study collected information on 20,158 people 18 years or older who visited the office of one of 3,439 physicians in three cities (Chicago, Los Angeles, and Boston) during a 9-day period in 1987. Data on the prevalence of hypertension, diabetes, and congestive heart failure (CHF) were collected from physician-completed encounter forms. Patients were classified as belonging to one of five systems of care for comparison purposes: HMO, multispecialty group-prepaid, multispecialty group-fee for service, solo practice or small single-specialty group-prepaid, or solo practice or small single-specialty group-fee for service. Kravitz et al. (1992) found that patients in the last group were more likely to report the presence of a chronic condition (62%) than patients in the other groups, with the lowest prevalence occurring in the multispecialty prepaid group (49.7%). These two groups also exhibited the greatest difference in number of chronic conditions per patient (1.10 versus 0.69) and in prevalence of each of the three chronic conditions noted above. The HMO group was lower than the solo fee-for-service group as well, but not as dramatically. Although the comparisons by Kravitz et al. are relatively comprehensive, their study does have limitations. For instance, they express concerns about the national representativeness of their sample, cautioning that "the results should probably not be generalized beyond the three cities studied" (p. 1622). Also, their data were collected during a time when patients enrolled in MCOs were in the minority, particularly in Boston and Chicago. It is not clear whether the differences they found would continue in the present, when a much larger proportion of the population is served by these types of organizations.

A study by Taylor, Beauregard, and Vistnes (1995) addressed the national representativeness issue by using data collected as part of the National Medical Expenditure Survey conducted in 1987. This survey is based on a random sample of adults in the United States. The authors compared the characteristics of 3,750 people enrolled in HMOs versus 18,079 enrolled in fee-for-service programs. Although the HMO enrollees were significantly younger, there was no significant difference in the percentage with three or more chronic conditions, in unadjusted comparisons. The percentages of people in HMOs with diabetes and with cardiovascular diseases were lower, but there were no significant differences for hypertension or arthritis. When adjustments were made for differences in demographic characteristics between the two groups, none of the comparisons were statistically significant. This suggests that, for the two conditions (diabetes and cardiovascular disease) where differences were significant in unadjusted comparisons, HMOs had a lower percentage because their enrollees were younger, not because they enrolled a healthier population at any given age. The authors conducted a sensitivity analysis that suggested these results were not influenced by whether or not the person had a choice of health plan at the time of enrollment. One important feature to note regarding the Taylor et al. study is that they used self-reported measures, as opposed to data abstracted from provider records or reports. This could introduce error in the identification of the presence of a specific chronic illness, but there is probably no reason to think that this error occurs more frequently in a particular direction among HMO versus fee-for-service enrollees. Therefore, their comparisons are not likely to be affected. Moreover, the Taylor et al., study results are more likely to be generalizable to the national population than the Dowd and Feldman (1985) or the Kravitz et al. (1992) findings. However, Kravitz et al. used a more sophisticated categorization scheme for their study participants. As with Kravitz et al., care must be taken in generalizing the Taylor et al. results to the present population nationwide because of the growth in managed care enrollment since 1987.

This problem was somewhat ameliorated in a study by Fama, Fox, and White (1995), who used data collected as part of the 1992 National Health Interview Survey. This survey was targeted at the noninstitutionalized population under the age of 65. These authors contrasted the self-reported presence of chronic illness among 40,956 people covered by indemnity insurance versus 19,575 in HMOs. They identify their most striking finding as "how little HMOs and indemnity plans differ in the prevalence of chronic conditions" (p. 237). They found no significant differences in comparisons using adjusted and unadjusted data. As a result, they reach some fairly strong conclusions: "This analysis refutes the notion that chronic illness is more prevalent among nonelderly people covered by indemnity insurance than among those covered by HMOs" (p. 242). Their study leaves open, however, the question of whether differences exist in either the Medicare or Medicaid populations.

In a more recent but much more limited study, Cogswell, Nelson, and Koplan (1997) compared the presence of chronic conditions among 24,706 enrollees, 18 years and older, in Prudential HMO and point-of-service products in 1995 with 35,146 respondents to the Behavioral Risk Factor Surveillance System (BRFSS) surveys (administered by the states) in 1994, in the states where the Prudential products were also offered. The Prudential survey questions were worded in the same way as the BRFSS questions to facilitate comparisons, and a subgroup of BRFSS enrollees was defined that was privately insured. Although there were significant demographic differences between the two samples, unadjusted and adjusted prevalence rates for diabetes and hypertension were similar. The information on chronic conditions used by Cogswell et al. (1997) was restricted to hypertension and diabetes, and data were collected through two different surveys conducted by different entities, raising some questions about comparability of responses. Also, the MCO comparison group was drawn from a single insurer organization, which suggests caution in generalizing from the results.

Although these five studies all compared the chronic illness status of enrollees in MCOs to those in some form of indemnity insurance, using data collected from a variety of sources, only Dowd and Feldman (1985) found striking differences. The next strongest evidence that chronic illnesses may be more prevalent among fee-for-service enrollees was contained in the Kravitz et al. (1992) article based on data collected as part of the Medical Outcomes Study. However, in this study, the differences reported between patient groups in different fee-for-service practice settings (multispecialty group versus solo) are similar to differences between fee-for-service and HMO patients. And, as in the Dowd and Feldman study, these data are now 15 years old, raising questions about their current relevance, given the much higher enrollment in MCOs at present. Comparisons based on more recent data do not suggest that differences exist between MCO and fee-for-service populations. In summary, the empirical evidence concerning the prevalence of people with chronic illnesses in MCOs versus other arrangements is quite sparse but does not suggest that MCOs serve substantially fewer of these people, proportionately. There are virtually no national studies based on recent data or comparing enrolled populations in different types of MCOs. This would appear to be a fruitful area for new research studies.

Are more or fewer medical (and nonmedical) services sought and received by people with chronic illnesses in MCOs versus people in traditional insurance arrangements? Are there differences in use of specialists? How does the health status for people with chronic illness enrolled in MCOs compare to the status of similar people in traditional insurance arrangements?

The review of the literature findings pertaining to these questions is combined in this section of the chapter, because a number of the reviewed studies addressed multiple objectives. Summaries of the principal findings are contained in Table 3.1. The studies can be divided into two types. The first type uses some aggregate measure of chronic illness to identify individuals for MCO versus traditional insurance comparisons. Typically, an individual is identified as chronically ill if he or she has one or more of a list of chronic illnesses. The second type of study focuses on individuals with a specific chronic illness. For example, individuals with hypertension enrolled in MCOs might be compared with a similar group of individuals with hypertension enrolled in traditional insurance plans. We begin by reviewing the findings from the aggregate studies.

Aggregate studies. We found five studies that presented results at the aggregate (presence/absence of a chronic illness) level. The earliest study, published in 1987, was based on data collected from 1976 to 1981 as part of the RAND National Health Insurance Experiment. Individuals were randomly assigned to an HMO (Group Health of Puget Sound) or traditional insurance plans. These data were collected through self-administered questionnaires and physical examinations. The authors, Sloss et al. (1987), found no significant differences in the treatment of people with chronic illness.

The Medical Outcomes Study (described above) also examined treatment and medical outcomes for people with chronic illness. The research team found that patients in the study who had chronic conditions (hypertension, diabetes, myocardial infarction, and CHF) and who were enrolled in prepaid plans had fewer hospitalizations, but the probability they had visited a physician for care in a prior 6-month period was significantly greater, although the difference was small in size (Nelson et al., 1998). Looking at a group of chronically ill study participants defined in a slightly different way (recent myocardial infarction, diabetes, hypertension, or depression), the researchers found no difference in physical health outcomes, on average. However, when they examined subgroups of people, they found that elderly people in HMOs experienced greater declines in physical health status and that poor people with initial poor health status did worse in MCOs (Ware, Bayliss, Rogers, Kosinski, & Tarlov, 1996).

(text continues on p. 55)

Table 3.1 Principal Findings

Reference	
General Chronic Illness	
Sloss et al. (1987)	Data were collected from 1976 to 1981 as part of the National Health Insurance Experiment. Participants ages 14 to 62 were randomly assigned to a health maintenance organization (HMO) (Group Health of Puget Sound) or a fee-for-service insurance plan. A self-administered questionnaire was completed at enrollment and at end of participation. About half of participants at baseline and all at exit had physical examinations. There were no significant results favoring fee for service or the HMO in treatment of chronic illness.
Ware et al. (1996)	Baseline data were collected on Medical Outcomes Study patients from February to October 1986 with hypertension, non-insulin dependent diabetes mellitus (NIDDM), recent myocardial infarctions, and depressive disorders. Four-year follow-up data were collected on 70% of baseline respondents. Respondents were classified as being treated in prepaid groups, independent physician associations (IPAs), large multispecialty groups, and solo or small single-specialty practices. On average, people in all groups experienced similar changes in physical health. Elderly in HMOs were twice as likely to decline in physical health, and poor patients in initial poor health did worse in HMOs. The comparisons were not significant after 1 year but were significant after 4 years.
Fama & Bernstein (1997)	National Health Interview Survey (1992) data on medical services use by chronically ill, nonelderly in HMOs and indemnity insurance were compared, where chronic illness included arthritis, asthma, diabetes, heart disease, and hypertension, along with 13 other chronic conditions. HMO enrollees were more likely to have visited physicians in the previous year, but there was no difference in the average number of visits for those with one or more visits.

(Continued)

Table 3.1 (Continued)

Reference	
General Chronic Illness	
Nelson et al. (1998)	Data were collected from Medical Outcomes Study patients from 1986 to 1990, with the following chronic conditions: hypertension, diabetes, myocardial infarction, and CHF. The prepaid patients had 31% fewer hospitalizations, 15% fewer after adjusting for group differences. The probability of having a visit for care in any 6-month period was slightly but significantly greater among prepaid patients than among fee-for-service patients, and their number of visits was slightly but insignificantly greater.
Druss et al. (2000)	Data were collected through a mail survey of a random sample of employees in three large companies at six sites. Respondents were compared within three types of insurance: fee-for-service, prepaid group, and IPA. Within each group, respondents with a chronic illness were compared to all other respondents along a variety of dimensions of satisfaction. In fee-for-service, there was no difference in percentage dissatisfied. In IPAs, chronically ill people were more dissatisfied on 12 of 14 measures, whereas in prepaid groups, they were more dissatisfied on 10 of 14. Both healthy and chronically ill respondents had higher overall dissatisfaction in fee-for-service, but differences between healthy and chronically ill respondents were significant only in managed care plans.
Hypertension	
Epstein et al. (1986)	Patients were selected from internists in large fee-for-service group practices and two HMOs. All patients were 16 years or older, had uncomplicated hypertension, were under treatment with medication, and had two or more visits during the study period of January 1978 to December 1979. Data were from chart abstraction. The use of the two highest-profit tests (as perceived by fee-for-service physicians) was 50% higher in the fee-for-service group. Patients in the HMO group averaged 50% more visits.
Gravdal et al. (1991)	Patients drawn from a single primary-care practice were classified as public assistance, capitated HMO, and fee for service. Visits were examined from June 1984 to May 1985 for each type (25 to 30 patients per type). Fee-for-service patients had the lowest mean utilization and public assistance patients the highest.

Preston & Retchin (1991)	Elderly patients from four group-practice HMOs and four IPA-model HMOs were compared to fee-for-service patients using medical records data from January 1983 to March 1986. There were 349 hypertensive patients in the HMO group and 336 in the fee-for-service group. Medical history-taking was more thorough for the HMO patients. HMO patients, in their first visit, were more likely to have funduscopic evaluation and be referred for eye exams. They were also more likely to receive a range of other tests and had more conservative measures (e.g., dietary counseling) recommended more often.
Udvarhelyi et al. (1991)	Equal numbers of HMO and fee-for-service patients were randomly chosen from four group practices that were part of one network-model HMO. Data were collected by chart review from November 1985 to October 1987; patients had to be older than 30 years of age and under treatment for hypertension for at least 6 months prior to study intake. Hypertensive HMO patients had higher visit rates, but there was no difference in use of diagnostic tests. HMO patients were more likely to achieve blood-pressure control.
Greenfield et al. (1995)	Baseline data were collected on Medical Outcomes Study patients for February to October 1986; outcomes included physiological and functional status after 2 years, functional status after 4 years, and mortality after 7 years. Patients were excluded if younger than 18 years and if they had medical conditions that overwhelmed hypertension. Comparisons were HMO versus fee-for-service and IPA versus fee-for-service. There were no significant differences in mean outcomes including medication use and yearly outpatient visits. More patients in fee-for-service were treated by specialists.
Joint Pain/Rheumatitis/ Osteoporosis	
Lubeck et al. (1985)	Patients in Kaiser (northern California), Mid-Peninsula Health Service (emphasis on patient self-care), and fee-for-service were compared. Patients were volunteers, older than 55 years, completing self-administered questionnaires. Fee-for-service patients initiated more visits over 18 months, whereas Mid-Peninsular patients had more telephone consultations. Appointment waiting time was longer at Kaiser, but Kaiser patients were more satisfied with their premiums.

(Continued)

Table 3.1 (Continued)

Reference	
General Chronic Illness	
Yelin et al. (1986)	Patients with office visits selected from a random sample of rhemuatologists in northern California (1982 to 1983) completed telephone interviews at entry into the study and 1 to 2 years later. There were no differences over time in the change in the number of painful joints but a greater decline in the number of swollen joints among patients in managed care organizations (MCOs). There was no difference in work loss, death rates, or improvement in functional status.
Clement et al. (1994)	A random sample of 6,476 Medicare beneficiaries in HMOs and 6,381 in fee-for-service Medicare were interviewed by telephone in 1990. HMO enrollees with joint pain (n = 2,243) were more likely then fee-for-service enrollees with joint pain to have a physician visit and some medication prescribed. They were less likely to see a specialist, have follow-up recommended, and have progress monitored. HMO enrollees were more likely to report symptom improvement.
Yelin at al. (1996)	Comparisons are based on sample described in Yelin et al. (1986) and additional patients were selected from rheumatology practices in 1987, generating 6,984 person-years of observation on utilization and outcomes. There was no difference in the quantity of care used in any 1-year period or over 11 years, nor were there differences in other outcomes.
Ward et al. (1998)	Patients in managed care settings (57) were compared to patients in fee-for-service settings (125) over a long time period (1981 to 1994). Patients completed health assessment questionnaires every 6 months for an average of 10.3 years. No differences between the two groups were found in long-term health outcomes, treatments, and health care utilization.
Diabetes	
Retchin & Preston (1991)	Elderly patients from four group-practice HMOs and four IPA-model HMOs were compared to fee-for-service patients, using medical records data from January 1983 to March 1986. There were 158 diabetic patients in the HMO group and 134 in the fee-for-service group. The HMO group was more likely to have

	funduscopic examination and urinalyses, and patients in poor control were more likely to be referred to an ophthalmologist. But HMO patients were less likely to receive influenza vaccinations. There were no differences in treatment with insulin.
Greenfield et al. (1995)	Baseline data were collected on Medical Outcomes Study patients for February to October 1986; outcomes included physiological and functional status after 2 years, functional status after 4 years, and mortality after 7 years. There were no significant differences in NIDDM outcomes. A greater proportion of patients in fee-for-service and IPA-model plans were treated by subspecialists in comparison to patients in HMO plans.
Lee et al. (1998)	Patients with diabetes enrolled in the Medical Outcomes Study were asked if they had seen an ophthalmologist in the 6 months prior to their study enrollment. Of the 522 patients with completed data, 38% reported an ophthalmologist visit. Receiving care in a prepaid plan (versus fee for service) was not a significant variable in predicting an ophthalmologist visit.
Shatin et al. (1998)	Administrative data from 1992 to 1993 for two IPA-model HMOs, located in different states but both part of United Health Care, were employed in comparing service use by children covered by Medicaid versus children covered by employer insurance. Utilization rates were consistently higher for Medicaid children in both plans, but the patterns of differences across plans varied considerably by type of service. With respect to differences across plans in services used by children in the employer insurance group, one plan used considerably more laboratory services but far fewer hospital days.
Hofer et al. (1999)	Resource use was compared for diabetic patients drawn from three practice sites (a staff-model HMO, an urban university teaching clinic, and a group of private-practice doctors) from 1990 to 1993. The outpatient visit rate in the private practice clinics was significantly higher than in the HMO, whereas hospitalizations were higher for the urban teaching-clinic patients.

(Continued)

Table 3.1 (Continued)

General Chronic Illness	
Peptic Ulcer	
Krantz et al. (1982)	Kaiser Permanente of Southern California data for 1970 through 1980 on hospital discharges with a diagnoses of peptic ulcer were compared to U.S. data. Kaiser hospitalization rates and age-adjusted mortality rates were below national rates by a substantial amount. Over the study period, U.S. rates declined whereas Kaiser rates were stable.
Congestive Heart Failure	
Retchin & Brown (1991)	A sample of HMO Medicare beneficiaries was selected from four group-model HMOs and four IPA-model HMOs and compared to fee-for-service patients recruited from hospitals in the same areas. Patients who were newly hospitalized for CHF were included in the study, and data were abstracted from medical records. HMO patients were much more likely to have a follow-up visit within a week after discharge, and HMO providers were more likely to order serum potassium levels regularly. There were no other treatment differences.
Ni et al. (1998)	Patients discharged in Oregon in 1995 ages 65 and older with CHF were classified as managed care, Medicare, Medicaid, commercial/private insurance, self-pay, and others. Medicare managed care patients had significantly shorter length of stay than other Medicare patients and were more likely to enter the hospital through the emergency room.
Asthma	
Shatin et al. (1998)	Administrative data from 1992 and 1993 for two IPA-model HMOs, located in different states but both part of United Health Care, were employed in comparing service use by children covered by Medicaid versus those covered by employer insurance. Utilization rates were consistently higher for Medicaid children in both plans, with the pattern of differences also consistent with respect to differences across the two plans in services used by children in the employer insurance group. One plan used considerably more laboratory visits, home health visits, and office visits.

Using more recent (1992) data from the National Health Interview Survey, Fama and Bernstein (1997) reported that HMO enrollees with 1 or more of 13 chronic conditions were more likely to have visited physicians in the previous year. However, they found no difference in the average number of visits.

Druss, Schlesinger, Thomas, and Allen (2000) conducted a different set of comparisons using data from a random sample of employees from three large companies. They grouped these employees into three categories defined by insurance coverage: fee-for-service, prepaid group, and IPA-model HMO. Within each insurance grouping, the satisfaction levels were compared between people with and without chronic illness. The authors found that, within the fee-for-service group, there was no difference in satisfaction levels but that within each HMO group, people with chronic illness were much less happy with their care in comparison to other enrollees. Although the authors did not conduct statistical tests, the raw data indicate that satisfaction levels overall, for people with and without chronic illness, were much lower in the fee-for-service group than in either of the HMO groups.

In summary, in studies using aggregate definitions of chronic illness, there is no evidence of less outpatient use on the part of chronically ill people in HMOs and, in fact, a weak suggestion of greater use of outpatient care. Data from the Medical Outcomes Study indicate less use of inpatient care by chronically ill people, but this finding is difficult to interpret. It could suggest that chronically ill people in MCOs have restricted access to inpatient care, or it could mean that outpatient care is more effective in MCOs, reducing the need for inpatient care. Comparisons of health status do not yield significant differences, on average. However, elderly people in the Medical Outcomes Study, as well as poor people in poor initial health, fared worse in MCOs. These findings are based on data that are 14 years old, suggesting a need for updated research studies on these subpopulations of people with chronic illness.

Studies by type of chronic illness: In the Medical Outcomes Study, the results of comparisons of health status for people with chronic illness varied by sociodemographic characteristics. Results might also vary by the characteristics of an individual's chronic illness. We found 16 published studies that compared MCO versus traditional insurance enrollees, by specific type of chronic illness. Five of these studies related to hypertension. In research conducted using data from the late 1970s, Epstein, Begg, and McNeil (1986) discovered that use of high profit-margin tests (as perceived by fee-for-service physicians) was 50% higher in traditional insurance arrangements, whereas patients in an HMO group averaged 50% more visits in a given time period. Three subsequent studies of hypertensive enrollees were published, all using data collected during the mid to late 1980s. The Medical Outcomes Study research team found no significant differences in outcomes, including medication use and patient satisfaction, among chronically ill hypertensives under different insurance arrangements (Greenfield, Rogers, Mangotich, Carney, & Tarlov, 1995). Udvarhelyi, Jennison, Phillips, and Epstein (1991) found that HMO patients with hypertension had higher visit rates, but the researchers did not find any difference in the use of diagnostic tests. In their study, they concluded that HMO patients were more likely to achieve blood-pressure control. Preston and Retchin (1991) also reported somewhat favorable results for an HMO group of elderly patients. They found that medical history-taking was more thorough for the HMO patients. HMO patients also were more likely to receive a range of other tests and had more conservative measures (e.g., dietary counseling) recommended more often. The Preston and Retchin (1991) results are particularly important as they are based on patients drawn from eight different HMOs, four group-practice and four IPA-model plans. Their sample was not only geographically diverse but also had a significant representation from MCOs other than group- or staff-model HMOs.

Five studies have been published that compare enrollees with joint pain, rheumatitis, or osteoporosis, but three of these studies are based in the same location, northern California. In early research, Lubeck, Brown, and Holman (1985) compared patients in the Kaiser Health Plan of Northern California and in fee-for-service care with patients under treatment at Mid-Peninsular Health Service, a practice with emphasis on patient self-care. Appointment waiting times were longer at Kaiser, and there were more patient-initiated visits under the fee-for-service plan. However, the patients were volunteers, and there was significant potential for selection effects to have influenced these comparisons. Yelin, Shearn, and Epstein (1986) tracked, over 2 years, the experiences of patients drawn from a random sample of rheumatologists in northern California (1982-1983). They found no difference in the number of painful joints over time but a decline in the number of swollen joints among the MCO patients. There were no differences in other outcome measures. Yelin, Criswell, and Feigenbaum (1996) continued to follow these patients, along with patients selected from a new set of rheumatology practices in 1987. In total, they accumulated almost 7,000 person-years of observations on outcomes and utilization. Their analysis of these data yielded no differences in utilization or outcomes. The length of the follow-up period makes this study unique among the comparative studies reviewed in this chapter. Finally, Clement, Retchin, Brown, and Stegall (1994) compared elderly HMO and traditional insurance (Medicare) enrollees with joint pain, using data collected through telephone interviews. They found that the HMO enrollees were more likely to have a physician visit and a prescribed medication. However, HMO enrollees were less likely to see specialists, have follow-up recommended, and be monitored. Taken together, the results of these studies demonstrate little difference in service use or outcomes for MCO versus traditional insurance patients with joint problems, although the Clement et al. (1994) results do suggest possible differences in treatment approaches.

Given the relative prevalence and importance of diabetes as a chronic illness, it is somewhat surprising that only four studies have compared the experience of diabetics in MCOs versus those with traditional insurance arrangements. The earliest study, conducted by Retchin and Preston (1991), was part of the same research project as the Preston and Retchin (1991) hypertension study described above. In comparing elderly HMO enrollees with diabetes to a similar group of patients in traditional insurance plans, Retchin and Preston found that tests were more likely to be administered to HMO patients and that HMO patients were more likely to be referred to ophthalmologists but less likely to receive influenza vaccinations. They concluded that "Medicare HMOs appear to provide at least equal quality of care for diabetes when compared with that received by similar patients in [fee for service] settings" (p. 2248). However, there were several limitations in their approach, which they acknowledged, including the lack of control for disease severity and the absence of comparisons of glycemic control.

A second important analysis was based on Medical Outcomes Study data. Greenfield, Rogers, Mangotich, Carney, and Taylor (1995) found that a greater proportion of patients in fee-for-service plans and

IPA-model plans were treated by subspecialists, as compared to patients in group-model plans, but they found no significant difference in patient outcomes for any of their measures. Lee et al. (1998) also used the Medical Outcomes Study data in their research but focused on visits to an opthamologist in the 6 months prior to enrollment into that study. They found no difference between prepaid and other study participants in the probability of an opthamologist visit.

Shatin, Levin, Ireys, and Haller (1998) also addressed care for patients with diabetes in MCOs, focusing on people 18 years old or younger enrolled in two United Health Care HMOs. They contrasted service utilization for Medicaid and privately insured enrollees in each HMO, reporting that Medicaid enrollees in each case had greater use. Although this was not emphasized in their analysis, the two HMOs appeared to use different approaches to treatment for the privately employed groups, particularly relating to laboratory services and inpatient care.

Hofer et al. (1999) studied the reliability of performance measures used in profiling physicians. They based their analysis on data collected from 1990 to 1993 as part of the Diabetes Patient Outcomes Research Team Study. In pursuing their main study objective, the authors calculated use rates for patients of a staff-model HMO, an urban university teaching clinic, and a group of private-practice physicians. They compared these rates on an unadjusted basis and also adjusted for age/sex and for case mix. In all three comparisons, outpatient visit rates were significantly greater for private-practice patients than for HMO patients. Hospitalization rates were similar for these two groups on the first two comparisons, but private-practice rates were significantly higher after case-mix adjustments. Hospitalization rates for the urban teaching clinic patients were much higher than for the other two groups.

There have been only two published studies relating to comparisons of CHF patients. Retchin and Brown (1991), under the same research project as described in Preston and Retchin (see hypertension above), examined patients newly hospitalized for CHF using medical records data. HMO patients were more likely to have a follow-up visit a week after discharge, and HMO providers were more likely to order serum potassium levels regularly, but no other differences were observed. This more aggressive outpatient-treatment profile for HMO patients is consistent with research evidence that suggests aggressive outpatient care can reduce or delay rehospitalizations and overall costs of care. HMOs that are at financial risk for all treatment costs have a financial incentive to pursue this approach.

One study relating to the management of peptic ulcers was reviewed. In this study, hospital discharge data at Kaiser Permanente of Northern California from 1970 and 1980 were compared to data for the United States as a whole. Kaiser hospitalization rates and age-adjusted mortality rates were substantially below U.S. averages, but U.S. rates declined whereas Kaiser rates were stable during the study period (Kurata, Honda, & Frankl, 1982). The present usefulness of these findings is diminished by the lack of a well-defined comparison group and by the early time period of the study.

Surprisingly, we also found only one study relating to asthma care, and this effort contrasted care across two MCOs, rather than comparing MCOs and traditional insurance. Shatin and colleagues (1998) found similar results to those reported above in their study of diabetes care; that is, considerable differences across the two study HMOs in the relative amounts of different services used to treat children with asthma.

In general, the findings for comparison studies involving specific chronic diseases are similar to the findings for studies that used aggregate chronic illness measures. The number of published articles in this area is relatively small, with several of the articles building on the same research projects. The data are now 10 to 15 years old or older, in most cases, and the research designs vary widely in their sophistication. The strongest conclusion that can be reached is that there seems to be no compelling evidence in the published research literature that enrollees in MCOs who have chronic illnesses receive less adequate service or have poorer outcomes than similar individuals in traditional insurance arrangements.

Discussion

In the literature comparing the experience of chronically ill individuals enrolled in MCOs versus those in traditional insurance plans, the majority of the studies do not find large differences. This should provide some reassurance for those who are concerned that people with chronic illness will fare worse in MCOs. However, in contrast to this general conclusion, there are a smaller number of studies where significant differences are found, and these studies raise important questions. For instance, Dowd and Feldman (1985) found that traditional insurance arrangements had a higher proportion of enrollees with chronic illnesses. Unfortunately, the data on which their study is based are more than 15 years old. It is not clear whether, at a time when most individuals receive care from MCOs, this finding would persist.

With respect to service use, the results of three related studies are of special note. First, Preston and Retchin's (1991) study of service use in the treatment of hypertension for Medicare enrollees is important because it is based on multiple HMOs, with both major model types represented, and it contains considerable detail regarding types of services used. Their results favored HMOs with respect to the taking of medical histories and the use of tests. Using the same research design, Clement and colleagues (1994) found that HMO enrollees were more likely to have an outpatient visit for treatment of joint pain, along with a prescribed medication, but they were less likely to see specialists, have follow-up recommended, and be monitored. Retchin and Brown (1991) conducted similar analyses for patients with CHF as did Retchin and Preston (1991) for patients with diabetes. These studies are relatively unique in this literature because they go beyond general measures of service use and are able to document different patterns of treatment for specific illnesses. The results suggest that care is delivered differently in HMOs for at least some people with chronic illnesses. However, much more research of this type needs to be done to understand the reasons for and implications of these different patterns of care.

Ultimately, the most important question is whether people with chronic illnesses fare better or worse in MCOs, from a health status viewpoint. The published literature is mostly inconclusive on this point, with the exception of the findings of Nelson et al. (1998), in an analysis conducted as part of the Medical Outcomes Study. They used an aggregate measure of chronic illness and found no overall difference in physical health status. However, when they analyzed the data by population subgroup, they found that the elderly and poor people with initially poor health status experienced greater declines in health status if they were in HMOs. This, of course, is exactly the fear expressed by some policy analysts, as discussed in Chapter 2. The findings of Nelson et al. (1998) suggest that further research in this area is needed. Although the study was published relatively recently, the data on which the results are based were collected a decade ago. Also, research is needed to determine if the significance of their findings varies by type of chronic illness.

In general, we found relatively few recent studies addressing the research questions stated at the beginning of the chapter. This may be because managed care has become so pervasive over the past decade that comparisons of managed care to traditional insurance no longer seem as policy relevant as they once were. However, we believe that the evolution of MCOs and changes in employer-benefit designs have created new avenues for comparative research. For instance, it is not known whether people with chronic illnesses fare differently in different types of MCOs. It also would be important to know if the answer varied with type of chronic illness or with other patient characteristics (e.g., age, income). Changes in employer-benefit designs that force employees to move from traditional plans into MCOs, when traditional plans are dropped entirely from benefit offerings, also raise interesting research questions. For instance, do people with chronic illnesses who are forced to move into MCOs experience associated declines in health status? Or does their health status improve? Again, knowing whether the answer varied by type of illness or personal characteristics would be important. And, how will recent and proposed changes in utilization management in some MCOs, which make it easier for chronically ill enrollees to directly access specialists, affect their health, relative to chronically ill enrollees in more restrictive MCOs? Continued research involving comparative studies done at the system level clearly is needed to address these and related questions.

References

Buchmueller, T. C., & Feldstein, P. J. (1997). The effect of price on switching among health plans. *Journal of Health Economics, 16,* 231-247.

Clement, D. G., Retchin, S. M., Brown, R. S., & Stegall, M. H. (1994). Access and outcomes of elderly patients enrolled in managed care. *Journal of the American Medical Association, 271*(19), 1487-1492. (Erratum in *Journal of the American Medical Association, 272*(4), 276; July 27, 1994)

Cogswell, M. E., Nelson, D., & Koplan, J. P. (1997). Surveying managed care members on chronic disease. *Health Affairs (Project Hope), 16*(6), 219-227.

Davidson, B. N., Sofaer, S., & Gertler, P. (1992). Consumer information and biased selection in the demand for coverage supplementing Medicare. *Social Science & Medicine, 34*(9), 1023-1034.

Dowd, B., & Feldman, R. (1985). Biased selection in Twin Cities health plans. *Advances in Health Economics and Health Services Research, 6*, 253-271.

Druss, B. G., Schlesinger, M., Thomas, T., & Allen, H. (2000, January/February). Chronic illness and plan satisfaction under managed care. *Health Affairs, 19*(1), 203-209.

Epstein, A. M., Begg, C. G., & McNeil, B. J. (1986, April 24). The use of ambulatory testing in prepaid and fee-for-service group practices. *New England Journal of Medicine, 314*(17), 1089-1094.

Fama, T., & Bernstein, A. (1997). A comparison of physician and hospital use among the nonelderly covered by HMOs and indemnity insurance. *Medical Care Research Review, 54*(2), 239-254.

Fama, T., Fox, P. D., and White, L. A. (1995). Do HMOs care for the chronically ill? *Health Affairs (Project Hope), 14*(1), 234-243.

Feldman, R., Finch, M., Dowd, B., & Cassou, S. (1989). The demand for employment-based health insurance plans. *The Journal of Human Resources, 24*(1), 115-142.

Gravdal, J. A., Krohm, C., & Glasser, M. (1991). Payment mechanism and patterns of use of medical services: The example of hypertension. *The Journal of Family Practice, 32*(1), 66-70.

Grazier, K. L., Richardson, W. C., Martin, D. P., & Diehr, P. (1986). Factors affecting choice of health care plans. *HSR: Health Services Research, 20*, 6.

Greenfield, S., Rogers, W., Mangotich, M., Carney, M. F., & Tarlov, A. R. (1995). Outcomes of patients with hypertension and non-insulin dependent diabetes mellitus treated by different systems and specialties: Results from the medical outcomes study. *Journal of the American Medical Association, 274*(18), 1436-1444.

Hellinger, F. J. (1995). Selection bias in HMOs and PPOs: A review of the evidence. *Inquiry, 32*(2), 135-142.

Hennelly, V. D., & Boxerman, S. B. (1983). Disenrollment from a prepaid group plan: A multivariate analysis. *Medical Care, 21*(12), 1154-1167.

Hofer, T. P., Hayward, R. A., Greenfield, S., Wagner, E. H., Kaplan, S. H., & Manning, W. G. (1999). The unreliability of individual physician "report cards" for assessing the costs of quality of care of a chronic disease. *Journal of the American Medical Association, 281*(22), 2098-2105.

Juba, D. A., Lave, J. R., & Shaddy, J. (1980). An analysis of the choice of health benefits plans. *Inquiry, 17*(1), 62-71.

Kravitz, R. L., Greenfield, S., Rogers, W., Manning, W. G., Jr., Zubkoff, M., Nelson, E. C., Tarlov, A. R., & Ware, J. E., Jr. (1992). Differences in the mix of patients among medical specialties and systems of care: Results from the medical outcomes study. *Journal of the American Medical Association, 267*(12), 1617-1623.

Kurata, J. H., Honda, G. D., & Frankl, H. (1982, November). Hospitalization and mobility rates for peptic ulcers: A comparison of a large health maintenance organization and United States data. *Gastroenterology, 83*, 1008-1016.

Lee, P. P., Meredith, L. S., Whitcup, S. M., Spritzer, K., & Hays, R. D. (1998). A comparison of self-reported utilization of ophthalmic care for diabetes in managed care versus fee-for-service. *Retina, 18*(4), 356-359.

Long, S. H., Settle, R. F., & Wrightson, C. W., Jr. (1988, October). Employee premiums, availability of alternative plans, and HMO disenrollment. *Medical Care, 26*(10), 927-938.

Lubeck, D. P., Brown, B. W., & Holman, H. R. (1985). Chronic disease and health system performance: Care of osteoarthritis across three health services. *Medical Care, 23*(3), 266-277.

McGuire, T. G. (1981). Price and membership in a prepaid group medical practice. *Medical Care, 19*(2), 172-183.

Merrill, J., Jackson, C., & Reuter, J. (1985). Factors that affect the HMO enrollment decision: A tale of two cities. *Inquiry, 22*(4), 388-395.

Nelson, E. C., McHorney, C. A., Manning, W. G., Jr., Rogers, W. H., Zubkoff, M., Greenfield, W., Ware, J. E., Jr., & Tarlov, A. R. (1998). A longitudinal study of hospitalization rates for patients with chronic disease: Results from the medical outcomes study. *Health Services Research, 32*(6), 759-774.

Ni, H., Nauman, D. J., & Hershberger, R. E. (1998). Managed care and outcomes of hospitalization among elderly patients with congestive heart failure. *Archives of Internal Medicine, 158*(11), 1231-1236.

Preston, J. A., & Retchin, S. M. (1991). The management of geriatric hypertension in health maintenance organizations. *Journal of the American Geriatric Society, 39*(7), 683-690.

Retchin, S. M., & Brown, B. (1991). Elderly patients with congestive heart failure under prepaid care. *The American Journal of Medicine, 90*(2), 236-242.

Retchin, S., & Preston, J. (1991). Effects of cost containment on the care of elderly diabetics. *Archives of Internal Medicine, 151*(11), 2244-2248.

Scanlon, D. P., Chernew, M., & Lave, J. R. (1997). Consumer health plan choice: Current knowledge and future directions. *Annual Review of Public Health, 18*, 507-528.

Shatin, D., Levin, R., Ireys, H. T., & Haller, V. (1998, October). Health care utilization by children with chronic illnesses: A comparison of Medicaid and employer-insured managed care. *Pediatrics, 102*(4), E44.

Short, P. F., & Taylor, A. K. (1989). *Premiums, benefits, and employee choice of health insurance options*. Rockville, MD: National Center for Health Services Research.

Sloss, E. M., Keeler, E. B. Brook, R. H., Operskalski, B. H., Goldberg, G. A., & Newhouse, J. P. (1987). Effect of a health maintenance organization on physiologic health: Results from a randomized trial. *Annals of Internal Medicine, 106*(1), 130-138.

Taylor, A. K., Beauregard, K. M., & Vistnes, J. P. (1995). Who belongs to HMOs: A comparison of fee-for-service versus HMO enrollees. *Medical Care Research Review, 52*(3), 389-408.

Udvarhelyi, I. S., Jennison, K., Phillips, R. S., & Epstein, A. M. (1991). Comparison of the quality of ambulatory care for fee-for-service and prepaid patients. *Annals of Internal Medicine, 115*(5), 394-400.

Ward, M. M., Lubeck, D., & Leigh, J. P. (1998). Long-term health outcomes of patients with rheumatoid arthritis treated in managed care and fee-for-service practice settings. *The Journal of Rheumatology, 25*(4), 641-649.

Ware, J. E., Jr., Bayliss, M. S., Rogers, W. H., Kosinski, M., & Tarlov, A. R. (1996). Differences in 4-year health outcomes for elderly and poor, chronically ill patients treated in HMO and fee-for-service systems: Results from the medical outcomes study. *Journal of the American Medical Association, 276*(13), 1039-1047.

Welch, W. P., & Frank, R. G. (1986). The predictors of HMO enrollee populations: Results from a national sample. *Inquiry, 23*(1), 16-22.

Wilensky G. R., & Rossiter, L. F. (1986, Spring). Patient self-selection in HMOs. *Health Affairs* (Project Hope), *5*(1), 66-80.

Yelin, E. H., Criswell, L. A., & Feigenbaum, P. G. (1996). Health care utilization and outcomes among persons with rheumatoid arthritis in fee-for-service and prepaid group practice settings. *Journal of the American Medical Association, 276*(13), 1048-1053.

Yelin, E. H., Shearn, M. A., & Epstein, W. V. (1986). Health outcomes for a chronic disease in prepaid group practice and fee for service settings: The case of rheumatoid arthritis. *Medical Care, 24*(3), 236-247.

4 The Prevalence of Chronic Illness Management Programs in Managed Care Organizations

In Chapter 3, we focused primarily on the research literature that compared the performance of managed care organizations (MCOs) in treating people with chronic illness to that of fee-for-service medicine. These comparisons were carried out at the organizational or system level. With a few notable exceptions, this research was not designed to assess the prevalence or effectiveness of specific strategies that have been used by MCOs to identify or treat people with chronic illnesses. In this chapter, we begin to address what is known about these strategies. We do this by reviewing and summarizing attempts in the literature to document the availability and diffusion of programs in MCOs targeted at enrollees with chronic illnesses. The objective is to determine, subject to the limitations of this literature, how widespread these programs are, which types of MCOs are likely to implement different types of chronic illness management programs, and if the prevalence of these programs is increasing or decreasing over time. We also intend that the literature review in this chapter will provide a context for the next two chapters. In Chapter 5, we discuss the use of administrative claims and medical records data by MCOs to support chronic illness treatment. Then, in Chapter 6, we examine the literature on the design and effectiveness of specific treatment approaches or models, implemented within a managed care framework, to address the needs of enrollees with chronic illnesses.

Background

As we noted in Chapter 2, the percentage of the population enrolled in MCOs has increased dramatically over the past decade. Most of this enrollment growth has occurred in newer models of MCOs that make use of broad provider networks, the building blocks of which are small primary-care and specialist physician practices. Physicians in these practices are linked to MCOs through contractual relationships and typically contract simultaneously with multiple MCOs. In their contracts, they agree to participate in various MCO initiatives that could affect the way in which they deliver care to their patients, including patients with chronic illnesses. In some cases, these initiatives involve the use of administrative and clinical data to assist physicians in tracking the receipt of services by patients and in reminding physicians when specific services should be delivered, according to benchmarks or treatment protocols. In other cases, the MCO may provide resources to assist physicians in managing the care of certain patients. These resources could include such things as educational programs for patients or nurse-based coordinated care programs targeted at patients with specific illnesses. In many, if not most, cases physicians can exercise discretion in their use of the information or programs made available to them by MCOs. In some cases, the MCO may provide the physician with a financial incentive to respond to the information provided by the MCO or to use the treatment program developed by the MCO. Although all MCOs are accountable for the care delivered to their defined populations of enrollees, typically, only a small portion of a physician's practice revenue derives from any single MCO. Thus, the MCO is not in a strong position to compel physicians to use the information or programs it provides for the treatment of enrollees with chronic illnesses. The situation within staff- or group-model HMOs is somewhat different. Here, the physician is a salaried employee of the staff-model plan or the group-practice sponsor of the HMO and has been inducted into the culture of the organization. Physicians in these plans are more likely to be involved in the development of chronic illness treatment initiatives and may be more likely to support their implementation. However, there are relatively few pure staff- or group-model HMOs still functioning, as most plans of this type have added contracting physicians to their networks in response to purchaser desires for a broader choice of physicians and for wider geographic dispersion of the HMO's network.

The metamorphosis that has occurred over the past decade in the structure of many MCOs, as well as the increase in the number of physicians in any given market who have contracts with multiple different MCOs, arguably has made it more difficult for MCOs to implement systemwide strategies to manage chronic illnesses. This suggests that, all else being equal, one would expect a decline in the number of MCOs investing scarce resources in the implementation of chronic illness management initiatives. Where initiatives are developed by MCOs, they will most likely be in areas where there is clear potential for short-term financial payoff (Shulkin, 1999). On the other hand, some market forces have pushed MCOs in the direction of more active management of enrollees with chronic illnesses. For instance, purchasers are increasingly demanding evidence that MCOs are actively trying to manage care in ways that enhance quality. And, accreditation through the National Committee on Quality Assurance requires that MCOs report data on their performance relative to population-based standards. As noted in Chapter 2, two of these standards relate to chronic illness treatment. Finally, if MCOs expand their penetration into the Medicare market, the number of enrollees with one or more chronic illnesses is likely to increase, which enhances the potential financial viability of some kinds of chronic illness management initiatives. These considerations suggest that the number of MCOs attempting to implement initiatives for managing chronic illness may be relatively high and, possibly, increasing.

In an attempt to determine the prevalence of MCO efforts to develop and implement initiatives directed at the treatment of enrollees with chronic illness, we searched the literature as described in Chapter 1. We found very few publications in this general area. In this chapter, we first briefly summarize the results of four studies, all of which are limited in their scope or relevance to our objectives. We then devote the rest of the chapter to a discussion of the two most significant efforts identified in our literature search: a survey of 69 organizations and 72 chronic illness management programs by Wagner, Davis, Schaefer, Von Korff, and Austin (1999) and two national surveys conducted by InterStudy (1996, 1997) that reported data on the implementation of these programs in HMOs.

Small-Scale Studies

We identified four somewhat limited studies of the development and implementation of chronic illness management programs in MCOs. Chronologically, the earliest of these studies was by Fox, Wicks, and Newacheck (1993). This study had as its general objective the assessment of how well HMOs met the needs of children with disabilities due to chronic conditions. As part of their research, the authors surveyed 95 geographically dispersed HMOs in 1989, with 59 responding. They collected information on basic benefits and referral policies and then evaluated these data to ascertain potential impact on the ability of children with chronic conditions to secure needed care. Their finding with the greatest relevance for this chapter is that HMOs were much more likely to provide medical case management as a covered benefit than a comparison group of traditional insurance plans but that "despite the touting of care coordination as an attribute of HMOs, relatively few plans provide case management that is comprehensive" (p. 552). The Fox et al. (1993) results have limited relevance for our purposes, in that they derive solely from an examination of HMO basic benefit coverages. Their survey did not ask directly about programs or initiatives under development or in place to serve people with specific chronic illnesses, nor did they ask about systemwide efforts to support chronic illness treatment.

A second small-scale study was focused on the disease management services provided by MCOs for the treatment of diabetes ("Big

Changes," 1998). Rather than collecting data from HMOs, this study relied on a survey of 252 large employers conducted by a commercial survey firm. The survey findings suggest that about two thirds of the health plans available to the employees of these firms do not cover patient education classes for members with diabetes, about 40% do not cover laboratory tests, and about 30% do not cover blood-glucose meters or an annual dilated eye examination. However, most plans did cover disease management services for insulin dependent (Type I) diabetics. The study results were not published in a peer-reviewed journal, and the funder for the study was a leading maker of blood-glucose meters. It is not clear how the employer sample was selected or what the response rate was for the survey.

A third set of relevant findings was disseminated as part of a report, *The State of Health Insurance in California, 1999,* which was prepared by the University of California, Berkeley, and the University of California, Los Angeles (Schauffler & Brown, 2000). This report contains 1998 data from a survey conducted in 1999 in which California HMOs were asked to report their disease management programs, both implemented and under development. Of the 25 HMOs surveyed, 15 reported that they had implemented asthma programs, and 4 reported that they had asthma programs under development. Thirteen HMOs reported diabetes programs, with 6 reporting programs under development, and 9 reported congestive heart failure (CHF) programs, with 5 reporting programs under development. Three or fewer HMOs reported having implemented programs for cholesterol, hypertension, arthritis, peptic ulcers, or osteoporosis. Of the HMOs with programs, most reported the use of protocols or guidelines, health care data, partnerships with other organizations, performance measures, and the training of primary-care physicians. None reported that they gave providers additional compensation for participating in the programs. About 88% of the HMOs with programs said that they tracked at least one outcome measure to evaluate program performance. More than half identified patient health status, number of inpatient stays, or patient satisfaction as measures they tracked. The California results are limited in their usefulness because they describe only HMO practices in California, where managed care has a longer history than in the rest of America. Also, little information is available concerning data collection, and the number of HMOs surveyed was relatively small.

A fourth study of interest focused on innovative programs for serving chronically ill older people (Boult, Kane, Pacala, & Wagner, 1999). The authors used an expert panel to identify programs that panel members believed to be "innovative and field tested." The directors of 31 programs then completed a 60-minute semistructured telephone interview to collect data on program origin, scope, operations, funding, and (when available) outcomes. Half of the programs were sponsored by HMOs and half by provider organizations. Several of the provider organizations participating in the survey were experienced in managed care contracts (e.g. Fairview, Minneapolis; Henry Ford Medical Group, Detroit; Intermountain Health, Salt Lake City; Carle Clinic, Champaign-Urbana). The authors found that, although these programs varied considerably in their origins and goals, "they tended to rely on 1 or more of 4 interrelated strategies—targeting high-risk seniors, using teams to provide care, shifting the site of care, and redesigning primary care" (p. 1169). The authors also noted the lack of rigorous evaluation of these and other programs designed to serve chronically ill seniors.

The Boult et al. (1999) study provides valuable comparative information about a select subset of programs serving seniors, an important subgroup of chronically ill people. However, the generalizability of the survey results to other MCOs and provider organizations with chronic illness management programs, or to other subgroups of the population, is questionable.

The Wagner et al. Study

Wagner et al. (1999) reported results of a study that is similar in design to the Boult et al. (1999) study but broader in its scope. These authors conducted telephone interviews with representatives from 72 programs housed in 69 different organizations. The programs were identified by a panel of experts in the field of chronic illness care as innovative or effective programs. The survey collected information on program components and on implementation and operational issues. The 72 surveyed programs represented 79% of the nominated programs. Most of the surveyed programs were located within a larger health care organization; about half of the programs were located in HMOs. The findings are not presented in a manner that permits them to be disaggregated by type of organization, but it seems safe to assume that most of the programs were implemented in some type of managed care environment. About half of the programs addressed multiple chronic conditions. For those that focused on single conditions, diabetes was the most common. About 58% of the programs actively identified and recruited patients, and 64% said that physician referral was an important source of patients. Primary care was an integral part of treatment in only about a third of the programs. Nurse specialists (50%), medical specialists (33%), and nurse or social work case managers (32%) were used relatively frequently in the treatment process. Fewer than 20% of the programs offered providers financial incentives for participation.

The authors gathered information about the presence of various structures and activities that are components of a Model for Effective Chronic Illness Care, which they describe in the article. They found that very few programs (18%) offered self-management support as a component, and then typically only where it was the primary program focus. Relative to usual methods for treating patients with chronic illnesses, most of the programs had greater involvement of nonphysicians in patient care and more aggressive follow-up of patients. More than 80% cited some form of case management, but this frequently focused on utilization management. About 60% of programs used specific practice guidelines, usually accompanied by some provider training. About half had updated their computer systems to facilitate program implementation, particularly in support of registries to identify patients and of reminder and feedback systems for providers.

Survey respondents identified enthusiastic, supportive organizational leadership as a key success factor. Physician resistance to changes in practice patterns and established clinical cultures was seen as a significant barrier. Providers pressed for time were likely to view any new initiative as making their situation worse, and this was a barrier to the use of chronic illness management programs. Changing organizational structures and staff turnover were seen as implementation barriers as well. Wagner and colleagues (1999) concluded that most programs "proved to be limited in their reach and effectiveness" (p. 65). About half could not identify the size of the population they were to serve. The authors also noted that "relatively few organizations have made the comprehensive system changes associated with demonstrably better patient and system outcomes" (p. 65).

The strength of this study is that, like Boult et al. (1999), it provides a relatively in-depth look at the way in which chronic illness management programs are implemented in health care organizations, with HMOs constituting about half of the organizations surveyed. In addition to documenting the components of the programs, the survey also addressed the factors that are facilitators and barriers to program implementation and operations. A primary limitation of the study relates to generalizability. The programs were selected because they were believed to be superior in design and/or performance. Therefore, they represented the best that had been achieved, but not necessarily the "typical" program. It would not be appropriate to generalize to all implemented chronic illness management programs based on the survey data in this article. Nevertheless, with this caution, the article provides a reasonably broad-based, yet in-depth view of operational chronic illness management programs.

The InterStudy Survey

InterStudy is an organization that tracks the development of the managed care industry, and especially the growth and evolution of HMOs. It does this through semiannual surveys of HMOs. The results of these surveys typically are not published in peer-reviewed journals but are widely circulated in the HMO industry. In the spring of 1996 and again in the spring of 1997, InterStudy included in its surveys a set of questions about the development and implementation of what it labeled *disease management programs.* In 1997, 282 of an eligible 609 HMOs (46% response rate) returned the portions of the questionnaire relating to disease management programs. Relative to the average HMO, the HMOs providing these data tended to be larger and older and were more likely to be an independent physician association (IPA) or network model and to be not-for-profit. The location of the respondents was representative of the location of all HMOs nationwide, and national HMOs, Blue Cross/Blue Shield, and independent HMOs were also proportionately represented among the respondents. A smaller proportion of HMOs (38%) responded to the disease management portion of the survey in 1996. As in 1997, larger plans were more likely to respond.

In its survey, InterStudy classified a wide range of programs as involving disease management, including many that addressed medical problems that do not meet our definition of *chronic* (e.g., high-risk pregnancy programs) or that we have excluded from our review for other reasons (e.g., depression; see Chapter 1). In this chapter, we discuss only the InterStudy survey findings that relate to the chronic illnesses that are the focus of this book. An interesting aspect of InterStudy's survey approach is that HMOs were asked to distinguish between programs that were implemented versus those that were in the developmental stage. As Table 4.1 indicates, in both 1996 and 1997, over half of the respondents reported that asthma and diabetes programs were under development. For most chronic illnesses, there was a small increase in the number of HMOs reporting programs under development between 1996 and 1997. Among the illnesses listed in Table 4.1, diabetes and asthma are the most prevalent in employed populations, the dominant source for HMO enrollment.

When asked for their expectations concerning the potential benefits of disease management programs, relatively few of the 1997 survey respondents said they expected these programs to reduce costs. Programs for peptic ulcer, osteoporosis, hypertension, and high cholesterol were seen by the majority of respondents as potentially cost-reducing. A minority of the respondents were of the opinion that diabetes, CHF, and asthma programs reduced costs, even though there is literature (see Chapter 6) suggesting these programs can generate cost savings, sometimes in the short term. However, the majority of respondents believed asthma, diabetes, and CHF programs improved processes of care and patient outcomes. The respondents also said that diabetes and asthma programs generated the greatest marketing benefits.

Figure 4.1, adapted from the InterStudy survey data, shows that HMOs typically develop two to three chronic illness management programs. Analyses of these data by InterStudy suggest that, in markets where HMOs enroll a larger percentage of the population, HMOs are likely to develop more disease management programs. InterStudy speculates that higher levels of HMO market penetration coincide with increased competitive pressure to control cost and to demonstrate care-

Table 4.1 Development of Disease-Management Programs in Health Maintenance Organizations (HMOs) (percentage of HMOs reporting program development, not implementation)

Condition	1996 n = 262	1997 n = 282
Asthma	61.5	65.9
Diabetes	58.4	62.8
Congestive heart failure	26.7	32.2
Hypercholesterolemia	20.2	22.1
Hypertension	17.9	16.3
Peptic ulcer	n/a	13.6
Osteoporosis	3.8	5.0
Arthritis	1.5	2.7

SOURCE: Data are from InterStudy, 1996, 1997.

improvement efforts to purchasers. Size of the HMO also explains a significant portion of the variation in the number of programs offered by an HMO, with larger HMOs implementing more programs.

Whereas Figure 4.1 displays the overall relative frequency with which chronic illness management programs are present in HMOs, Table 4.2 (adapted from InterStudy data) provides some indication of the order in which HMOs are likely to add these programs. Only 23 HMOs reported one program, but the data suggest that this program is most likely to focus on asthma management. Asthma and diabetes programs, both diseases with relatively high prevalence among HMO members, are likely to be available if an HMO offers two or more chronic illness management programs. In HMOs with three or more programs, CHF programs are likely to be present. The pattern of adoption is less clear for programs for peptic ulcers, osteoporosis, and arthritis.

The InterStudy survey data also provide some insight into the process used by HMOs to develop and implement programs for treating chronic illness. The majority of HMOs (69% of the 262 HMO respondents in 1996) report that it takes 6 months to 1 year to move a chronic illness management program from concept to implementation. Program

Chronic Illness Management 75

```
Percent of HMOs
                    33.7%   30.0%

         12.1%                     11.1%   10.0%
                                                    3.2%
           1      2      3      4      5      6
```

Number of Chronic Illness Programs Developed at HMOs
n=190

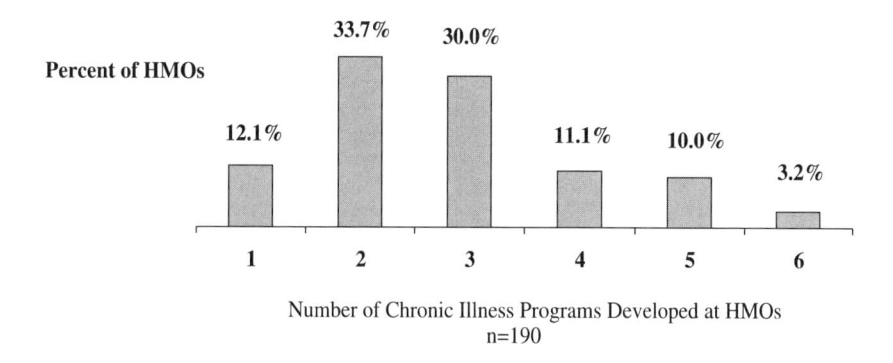

Figure 4.1. Multiple Chronic Illness-Management Programs at Health Maintenance Organizations
SOURCE: Adapted from InterStudy data, 1996, 1997.

development typically proceeds with medical directors, physicians, and nurses as part of a project team. HMO programs commonly involve the use of patient-level data (claims and other), training for primary- and specialty-care physicians, use of information systems, and partnering with other organizations. Program effectiveness is assessed by a wide range of measures, including changes in hospitalizations and lengths of stay, patient satisfaction as measured through patient surveys, clinical performance measures (e.g., rates of eye examinations for diabetics), changes in the utilization and costs of pharmaceuticals, ambulatory visits, diagnostic tests, patient health status, and overall system costs. Larger, physician group practice-based, not-for-profit HMOs are more likely to include changes in patient health status in their evaluations, in comparison with other HMOs.

In 1997, the gap between development and implementation of chronic illness management programs was the greatest for asthma and diabetes; more HMOs had developed but not implemented these programs (Figure 4.2), with a similar gap apparent for CHF. In analyses of their data, InterStudy found that several factors differentiated HMOs that had developed (but not implemented) programs from HMOs that had implemented programs (Table 4.3). HMOs that have implemented the three most common programs tend to be larger and more profitable (report smaller losses), less financially liquid, and more involved with Medicare. Both size and profit could be indicators of ability to invest in

Table 4.2 Percentage of Health Maintenance Organizations (HMOs) With Specific Chronic Illness-Management Programs, Given the Total Number of Chronic Illness-Management Programs in the HMO

	Number of Chronic Disease Programs					
	1	2	3	4	5	6
Number of HMOs	23	64	57	21	19	6
Asthma	73.9	79.7	89.5	85.7	94.7	100
Diabetes	13.0	87.5	91.2	85.7	100	100
Hypertension	4.3	3.1	10.5	38.1	78.9	100
Hypercholesterolemia	0.0	4.7	24.6	76.2	78.9	83.3
Congestive heart failure	4.3	14.1	66.7	57.1	78.9	66.7
Peptic ulcer	0.0	7.8	10.5	42.9	36.8	83.3
Arthritis	4.3	0.0	0.0	4.8	15.8	33.3
Osteoporosis	0.0	3.1	7.0	9.5	15.8	33.3

SOURCE: Data are from InterStudy, 1996, 1997.

and build new programs. Implementation of programs for asthma management is more likely in markets with greater competition, that is, where there are more HMOs and market penetration is higher. This suggests decisions regarding the implementation of these programs are affected, at least in part, by external market pressures. It is interesting to note that, for these chronic illnesses, HMO characteristics such as for-profit/not-for-profit, model type, and age of plan are not significantly different between developers and implementers. However, these characteristics are more often significant in comparing HMO implementers versus developers of less common chronic illness management programs (Table 4.4).

The InterStudy survey data provide a relatively broad view of chronic illness management programs in MCOs but suffer from three important limitations. First, they pertain only to HMOs. Other types of MCOs, such as PPOs, are not included in the InterStudy survey. We were not able to identify any comprehensive database that documented

Chronic Illness Management 77

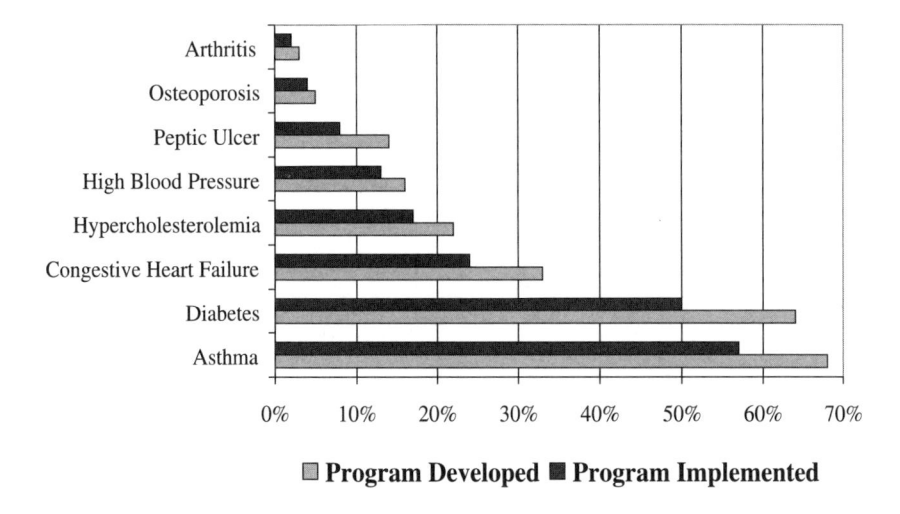

[Bar chart showing Program Developed and Program Implemented percentages for: Arthritis, Osteoporosis, Peptic Ulcer, High Blood Pressure, Hypercholesterolemia, Congestive Heart Failure, Diabetes, Asthma]

☐ **Program Developed** ■ **Program Implemented**

Figure 4.2. Development and Implementation of Chronic Illness Management Programs ($n = 282$)
SOURCE: Adapted from InterStudy data, 1996, 1997.

and tracked chronic illness management programs in other types of MCOs. However, in other research not specifically directed at chronic disease management, InterStudy learned that PPO involvement in chronic disease programs is very limited and is driven by employer demand for them.

A second limitation of the InterStudy surveys is that the data collected from the responding HMOs are of an overview nature; most details about program operations are unmeasured. Finally, and perhaps most important, it is not clear that the responding HMOs are representative of all HMOs. The respondents differ by some measurable characteristics, as noted above, but could very well differ in ways that are not easily observable. For instance, HMOs with disease management programs might be more likely to complete this portion of the InterStudy survey, whereas those without programs might see little value in doing so. If this were the case, the findings would overstate the prevalence of chronic illness management programs in HMOs. The less than 50% response rate for the disease management portion of the InterStudy survey raises this as a significant concern.

Table 4.3 Implementers Versus Developers of Common Chronic Illness Management Programs (1997)

Chronic Illness Management Program	Average HMO Developing But Not Yet Implementing Programs	Average HMO With Implemented Programs	Significance Level for Difference Between Groups (p value)
Asthma			
Number of HMOs	24	137	
Efficiency (administrative expense/total operating revenue)	22.9%	15.5%	***
Profitability	–9.0%	–2.5%	***
Liquidity (current assets/current liabilities)	1.42	0.97	**
Penetration of primary market	27.7%	35.5%	***
Number of HMOs in primary market	9.5	12.2	**
Diabetes			
Number of HMOs	37	118	
Total HMO enrollment	104,890	224,823	*
Medicare enrollment	4,993	18,442	**
Profitability	–7.4	–2.2	***
Liquidity (current assets/current liabilities)	1.19	0.94	**
Congestive Heart Failure			
Number of HMOs	24	55	
Medicare enrollment	6,978	28,337	**
Profitability	–7.5%	–1.3%	***
Total revenue per member per month	$123	$152	**
Primary market's 2-year rate of HMO enrollment growth 1996-1998	30.7%	15.5%	**

SOURCE: Data are from InterStudy, 1996, 1997.
*p = .10. **p = .05. ***p = .01.

Chronic Illness Management

Table 4.4 Implementers Versus Developers (but not yet implementers) of Less Common Chronic Illness Management Programs (1997)

Disease Management Program	Average HMO Developing But Not Yet Implementing Programs	Average HMO With Implemented Programs	Significance of the Difference Between Groups (*p* value)
Hypercholesterolemia			
Number of HMOs	13	40	
Percentage of HMOs where physicians are in group practices	61%	30%	**
Hypertension			
Number of HMOs	8	29	
Tax status for-profit	25%	59%	*
Index of competition in primary market	.59	.72	*
Peptic ulcer			
Number of HMOs	10	22	
Percentage of HMOs with physicians in group practices	10%	54%	**
Osteoporosis			
Number of HMOs	4	9	
Index of competition in primary market[a]	.85	.73	*
Arthritis			
Number of HMOs	3	4	
No significant factors			

SOURCE: InterStudy, 1996, 1997.

a. 1 = perfect competition (many plans with similar market shares), 0 = monopoly (one HMO serving the market)

*p = .10; **p = .05; ***p = .01.

Vendor Products and Chronic Illness "Carve-Outs"

Although the InterStudy (1996, 1997) survey reports whether HMOs have developed or implemented chronic illness management programs, the organizational mechanism of implementation for HMOs and other types of MCOs is not clear. Presumably, the majority of HMOs construct their programs internally. However, vendor-provided programs are becoming increasingly available to HMOs and other types of MCOs. One type of vendor-provided program is the chronic illness "carve out," under which the MCO contracts with an external organization to provide care. These sorts of programs offer possible advantages for MCOs. They could improve quality of care by concentrating the care of patients with a specific chronic illness in provider organizations that specialize in treating that illness. Organizations accepting carve-out contracts would have a strong incentive to develop treatment approaches that measurably improve patient outcomes while containing treatment costs. A concern about carve-out contracts between MCOs and independent organizations is that they could have a negative impact on coordination of care, resulting in unnecessary and costly duplication of services between MCO providers and carve-out firms. Managing the coordination of care could be challenging for MCOs and potentially frustrating for providers in MCO networks.

There is some information about the prevalence of behavorial health care carve-out relationships between MCOs and contracting firms. However, there does not appear to be similar information about carve-out arrangements for chronic illnesses such as diabetes and asthma. This may be because these arrangements are relatively infrequent. Blumenthal and Buntin (1998) observe,

> Accounts in the business and employee benefits literature would lead readers to think that carve-outs and disease management programs are widespread. However, a close reading reveals that although many of these programs are under development, few (other than managed behavioral health and managed pharmacy programs) have actually been sold to employers or managed care companies. (p. SP48)

According to Blumenthal and Buntin (1998), "It appears that purchasers have been unwilling to fragment responsibility for their patients' care or to restrict patients to networks created by carve-out entities" (p. SP48).

To date, vendor products have focused primarily on diabetes and asthma management, although some products offer management strategies for other conditions as well. Vendor products are available for purchase from organizations such as Pharmacy Benefits Managers (PBMs), from corporations dedicated solely to providing disease management products and, in a few cases, from health care organizations (such as the International Diabetes Center of HealthSystem Minnesota or the Lovelace Health System). Typically, products offered by PBMs focus on the analysis of pharmacy data, sometimes in combination with medical claims data. These products usually emphasize assessment of current practices rather than implementation of patient-care initiatives. Products created by disease management corporations and by individual care centers tend to offer both assessment of current practices and specific patient-care initiatives.

Vendor Products for Use With Multiple Diseases

Lovelace Health System of Albuquerque, New Mexico, has developed the Episodes of Care (EOC) disease management strategy and, together with Greenstone Healthcare Solutions (a subsidiary of Pharmacia & Upjohn), markets the product to external organizations. An EOC is defined as all of the services provided to a patient with a particular medical problem within a defined time period. Each type of episode has an EOC team that includes specialists, primary-care physicians, nurse care managers, education specialists, and quality-measurement specialists. The EOC teams are responsible for developing care protocols and practice guidelines for their target episode. The goal of the EOC method is to reduce inappropriate care, improve system performance, and improve customer satisfaction. A total of 30 EOC units are planned, although as of 1997, the product had been launched only for diabetes, asthma, depression, and birth. To date, no evaluation of the EOC strategy outside of the Lovelace system is available, and only (that we could identify) the diabetes EOC has been formally evaluated in the peer-reviewed literature (see Chapter 5).

Vendor Products for Specific Chronic Illnesses

Staged Diabetes Management (SDM), developed by the International Diabetes Center at HealthSystem Minnesota, is one of the most widely known diabetes management interventions in the United States and internationally. SDM is designed for the care of diabetic patients in primary-care settings and emphasizes aggressive management of diabetes with patients as partners in their diabetes care (Mazze, Bergenstal, & Ginsberg, 1995). The cornerstone of the SDM program is a set of Decision Paths© and Road Maps©, care protocols that instruct providers on medication dosing and other aspects of diabetes management. These protocols detail, for example, the types of insulin or hypoglycemic agents, frequency, and dosing to be used. In the SDM system, patients move through various stages of diabetes management. If glycemic goals are not achieved by patients in a relatively timely fashion, patients are moved to a different management stage with an alternative approach for medication management, exercise, and meal planning (Mazze et al., 1995). With the help of SDM facilitators, program sites tailor the care protocols to suit their patient populations (Mazze et al., 1994, 1995). A version of SDM that is adaptable to new care systems is available (Mazze et al., 1995). For technologically advanced systems, SDM is available in an integrated, Windows-based computerized version (Ginsberg, Tan, Mazze, & Bergelson, 1998).

Testing of the SDM protocol has occurred in several sites across the United States and internationally since 1988. The results of a comparison of SDM-managed patients to usual-care patients revealed a 2% decrease in HbA1c levels among intervention group patients. Usual-care patients experienced no drop in HbA1c levels (Mazze et al., 1994). The pooled results of six sites implementing the program identified a 1.5% to 2.0% drop in HbA1c levels over a 12-month period, results comparable to those achieved in the Diabetes Control and Complications Trial (DCCT) (Ginsberg et al., 1998).

Diabetes NetCare is a comprehensive disease management program designed by the Diabetes Treatment Center of America for implementation in MCOs (Rubin, Dietrich, & Hawk, 1998). It provides management of diabetic populations patterned after the DCCT. NetCare profiles an organization's diabetic population, costs, and utilization, then tailors a management program to the particular MCO. Management includes coordination of care between physicians, hospitals, and other care providers. In addition, NetCare stratifies the diabetic population into severity levels and focuses resources on the most severe cases. All patients are assigned to a diabetes case manager and are taught diabetes self-management skills. Patients with elevated HbA1c levels are assigned to a complex-case manager, who more intensely manages care. NetCare provides the purchasing MCO with on-site administrative, clinical, and provider support and an electronic tracking system.

Rubin et al. (1998) describe the implementation of Diabetes NetCare in seven HMOs nationally with a total of more than 7,000 diabetic patients and evaluate indicators of improvements in care processes over a period from 9 to 12 months, depending on the HMO. Overall, frequency of annual HbA1c increased from 34% to 76% in the pooled population. Frequency of retinal exams, foot exams, and cholesterol screenings among diabetic patients also increased substantially across all organizations. Decreases in the number of hospitalizations, average hospital length of stay, and the total costs of care were observed for the diabetic populations of the HMOs (Rubin et al., 1998). A slight decrease in HbA1c levels across all plans was reported, but given nonstandardization of the test across laboratories, this decrease was not clinically meaningful.

MedImpact Pharmaceutical Management, Inc., a San Diego-based PBM, offers an asthma management product that emphasizes physician profiling (DaSilva, 1996). Using merged pharmaceutical and medical data, MedImpact identifies physicians who are "most and least efficient at managing asthma" and locates "thought leaders" (i.e., physicians whose patients' claims provide evidence that the physician has responded to asthma-care guidelines). Physicians are profiled according to total expenditures per asthma patient per year, the ratio of outpatient appointments relative to time since acute episode, steroid to beta-agonist ratio, emergency room (ER) visit to outpatient visit ratio, and frequency of specialist referral. Physician profiling is intended by MedImpact to serve as learning tool for physicians (DaSilva, 1996).

Diversified Pharmaceutical Services (DPS), a Minneapolis-based PBM, offered a number of asthma disease management products to

MCOs (DPS has since merged into Express Scripts). MacKinnon, Flagstad, Peterson, & Mesch-Beatty (1996) describe a partnership between DPS, the University of Wisconsin Hospital and Clinics, and U-Care, the university-sponsored HMO. A disease management program for asthma was developed for U-Care using administrative databases. Utilization rates in the HMO were compared to a set of asthma clinical guidelines developed by DPS. Profiles of patients using extremely high doses of medications were provided to network pharmacists, who offered counseling to patients regarding medication and peak-flow meter use (MacKinnon et al., 1996). The impact of the intervention on patient health outcomes was not reported.

DPS was also involved in a cooperative asthma management effort with Mid-Atlantic Medical Services, Inc. (an IPA-network HMO), and Integrated Therapeutics Group (the health maintenance subsidiary of Schering-Plough). The management strategy used administrative and pharmacy claims in combination with a patient survey to assess the impact of multiple asthma-education efforts (Buchner et al., 1998). Representatives from the Integrated Therapeutics Group provided physicians with asthma-treatment education based on National Heart, Lung, and Blood Institute guidelines. Physicians also were supplied with Asthma Kits (peak-flow meters, diaries, videos, and written information) to provide to their patients. Patients were identified for educational intervention by the appearance of adverse events in their claims information. Evaluation from 1 year prior to 1 year after intervention found improvements in health-related quality of life and patients' perceptions of the quality of the asthma self-management instruction they received. The intervention also resulted in a 30% increase in the number of asthmatic patients receiving inhaled corticosteroid therapy. The proportion of asthmatics with one or more visits to the ER remained unchanged following the intervention, although the proportion of patients with multiple hospitalizations decreased significantly, as did the rate of hospitalizations in the population (Buchner et al., 1998).

A community-pharmacy model for asthma care was designed by Family PharmaCare Center, Inc., in West Lafayette, Indiana, for marketing to MCOs (Rupp, McCallian, & Sheth, 1997). PharmaCare's program, AIM: Asthma Integrated Management, is a disease-state management intervention that focuses on education for pediatric asthma patients, particularly those with poorly controlled asthma. In pilot-testing, PharmaCare was paid a flat fee per patient referred by a physician in the participating HMO. Enrolled patients attend six scheduled educational appointments with pharmacists and asthma management educators. PharmaCare did not dispense medication to the patients from the pilot HMO, because the HMO had an exclusive contract with a pharmacy. This situation led to disenrollment in the program because it was not offered at the patients' pharmacy and was not necessarily convenient for patients. Outcomes information from the pilot-test of the PharmaCare intervention have not been published. Currently, PharmaCare is planning to expand the program to include diabetes, dyslipidemia, and hypertension management (Rupp et al., 1997).

For several reasons, it is difficult to assess the impact that vendor products have had on MCOs' ability to manage chronically ill patients based on the existing literature. First, the impact of the various types of vendor products on health outcomes or costs of care is largely unknown. The majority of articles that discuss the use of vendor products by MCOs appear in non–peer reviewed industry publications. Typically, they describe vendor products in great detail but do not present results from rigorous evaluations of the impact on patient health outcomes or costs of care (see Buchner et al., 1998, Rubin et al., 1998).

Second, in addition to a lack of information regarding the impact of these products on health outcomes and costs of care, there is limited information regarding the short- and long-term costs of the products themselves. Staged Diabetes Management, according to its designers, will achieve a break-even point (where costs saved due to the implementation of the program match the costs invested in the program) after 6 to 8 years. However, we found no peer-reviewed study that established a foundation for this claim. Rubin et al. (1998) assert that the Diabetes NetCare program breaks even when about 1,200 diabetic patients are enrolled per year. However, the proprietary nature of the NetCare program prevented Rubin et al. (1998) from publishing exact program costs. Although Buchner et al. (1998) evaluated the impact of their asthma management program on health outcomes and quality of life, they did not provide a discussion of program costs. Given that few descriptions of vendor products in the literature provide evaluations of health outcomes, it is not surprising that fewer still offer a detailed accounting of the costs of implementing these programs.

Third, physician acceptance of vendor products for disease management has not been studied. It is unclear, particularly in decentralized MCOs such as IPA networks, to what degree physicians accept an external program to manage care for their chronically ill patients or how well vendor products have managed to integrate physicians into their programs. DaSilva (1996) describes a program with almost exclusive focus on physician profiling, using administrative data. In addition to a lack of information regarding patient health outcomes, DaSilva (1996) does not provide a discussion of physician reaction to this program. In a discussion of Diabetes NetCare, Rubin et al. (1998) report that "85% of physicians thought the program provided better care to patients" (p. 2639). However, only 27% of physicians contacted responded to the satisfaction survey from which this information was drawn, and we can only assume that Rubin et al. (1998) are referring to 85% of the 27% who responded. This leaves a great deal of uncertainty regarding the true nature of physician acceptance of the program.

Discussion

The overwhelming conclusion from the review of the literature in this chapter is that very little information exists to document the prevalence of chronic illness management programs in MCOs, the structure of these programs, or the way in which they have been implemented. We were able to find no literature that addressed trends in prevalence over time, with the exception of the 1996 InterStudy survey that was repeated in 1997, a time period too short to provide useful trend data. The two most significant efforts in this area—the Wagner et al. (1999) article and the two InterStudy reports—each provide pieces of the overall picture. Wagner, Austin, and Von Korff (1996) focused on chronic illness management programs that are believed to be effective. By design, they did not attempt to document overall prevalence of programs or to report on "average programs." In their article, it is not entirely clear which programs were carried out in managed care settings. InterStudy focused on a particular type of MCO, the HMO. The generalizability of

InterStudy's survey findings is limited by the possibility that nonrespondents may have been HMOs that were less likely to have programs. There is virtually no information on the degree to which MCOs rely on vendor-developed products or chronic illness carve-outs to address the needs of members with specific chronic illnesses. In summary, this is an area of research that has been underexplored. There is little existing information on which to base an assessment of the prevalence of chronic illness management programs in managed care settings, how programs vary across types of MCO, or how they have changed over time.

References

Big changes for diabetes management. Is your MCO missing the boat? (1998, February). *Managed Care Strategies, 6*(2), 16, 21-22.

Blumenthal, D., & Buntin, M. (1998, June 25). Carve outs: Definition, experience, and choice among candidate conditions. *American Journal of Managed Care, 4,* SP45-SP57.

Boult, C., Kane R., Pacala, J., & Wagner, E. (1999, September). Innovative health care for chronically ill older persons: Results of a national survey. *The American Journal of Managed Care, 5*(9), 1162-1172.

Buchner, D. A., Butt, L. T., De Stefano, A., Edgren, B., Suarez, A., & Evans, R. M. (1998). Effects of an asthma management program on the asthmatic member: Patient-centered results of a 2-year study in a managed care organization. *American Journal of Managed Care, 4*(9), 1288-1297.

DaSilva, R. V. (1996). A disease management case study on asthma. *Clinical Therapeutics, 18*(6), 1374-1382.

Fox, H. B., Wicks, L. B., & Newacheck, P. W. (1993, Fall). State Medicaid health maintenance organization policies and special-needs children. *Health Care Financing Review, 15*(1), 25-37.

Ginsberg, B. H., Tan, M. H., Mazze, R., & Bergelson, A. (1998). Staged diabetes management: Computerizing a disease state management program. *Journal of Medical Systems, 22*(2), 77-87.

InterStudy. (1996, September). *Competitive edge* (Version 6.2, pp. 71-83). Bloomington, MN: Author.

InterStudy. (1997, October). *Competitive edge* (Version 7.2, pp. 63-72). Bloomington, MN: Author.

McGlynn, E. (1996, Summer). Choosing chronic illness measures for HEDIS: Conceptual framework and review of seven clinical areas. *Managed Care Quarterly, 4*(3), 54-77.

MacKinnon, N. J., Flagstad, M. S., Peterson, C. R., & Mesch-Beatty, K. (1996). Disease management program for asthma: Baseline assessment of resource use. *American Journal of Health System Pharmacy, 53*(5), 535-541.

Mazze, R. S., Bergenstal, R., & Ginsberg, B. (1995). Intensified diabetes management: Lessons from the diabetes control and complications trial. *International Journal of Clinical Pharmacology and Therapy, 33*(1), 43-51.

Mazze, R. S., Etzwiler, D. D., Strock, E., Peterson, K., McClave, C. R., Meszaros, J. F., Leigh, C., Owens, L. W., Deeb, L. C., & Peterson, A. (1994. Staged diabetes management: Toward an integrated model of diabetes care. *Diabetes Care, 17*(Suppl 1), 56-66.

Rubin, R. J., Dietrich, K. A., & Hawk, A. D. (1998). Clinical and economic impact of implementing a comprehensive diabetes management program in managed care. *Journal of Clinical Endocrinology and Metabolism, 83*(8), 2635-2642.

Rupp, M. T., McCallian, D. J., & Sheth, K. K. (1997). Developing and marketing a community pharmacy-based asthma management program. *Journal of the American Pharmaceutical Association, NS37*(6), 694-699.

Schauffler, H., Brown, E. (2000, January). *The state of health insurance in California, 1999.* Berkeley: Regents of the University of California.

Shulkin, D. (1999, April). Understanding the economics of succeeding in disease management. *Managed Care Interface,* pp 98-100, 102-104.

Wagner, E. H., Austin, B. T., & Von Korff, M. (1996). Organizing care for patients with chronic illness. *Milbank Quarterly, 74*(4), 511-544.

Wagner, E., Davis, C., Schaefer, J., Von Korff, M., & Austin, B. (1999, Summer). A survey of leading chronic disease management programs: Are they consistent with the literature? *Managed Care Quarterly, 7*(3), 56-66.

5 Use of Administrative and Medical Records Data by MCOs for Chronic Illness Management

The use of administrative claims and medical records data by managed care organizations (MCOs) to identify, within their defined population of enrollees, subgroups of individuals with specific chronic illnesses and to monitor clinic or systemwide care for these patients appears to be common in MCOs. Individual MCOs or groups of MCOs have been evaluated, or have evaluated themselves, relative to internal and industrywide benchmarks or clinical care guidelines. MCOs also have used administrative and medical records data to identify opportunities for quality improvement in their care for patients with chronic illnesses. These evaluations, whether or not they are published in the peer-reviewed literature, can provide important information about how MCOs provide care to people with chronic illnesses. Indeed, it is likely that most analyses of this type conducted by MCOs are not published in peer-reviewed journals, but instead are used internally as tools to inform quality improvement. In this chapter, we focus on the subset of studies that have been published in the peer-reviewed literature and for which MCOs have used administrative claims or medical records data to assess existing approaches to chronic illness management. In most cases, the studies did not indicate whether these MCOs subsequently developed management interventions based on their findings. It is likely that we have not identified all such studies through our literature search, as the terminology used to describe their subject matter is highly variable and they are published in an eclectic mix of journals. Therefore, our review is more illustrative than it is comprehensive.

Administrative claims and medical records data are used to achieve six general (and frequently overlapping) goals:

1. Benchmarking
2. Assessment of quality of existing care
3. Identification of opportunities for improvements in care
4. Profiling of clinics and providers
5. Characterization of high-risk patients
6. Simulation of possible disease management interventions

Analyses of chronic disease management practices within organizations using administrative claims and medical records data take advantage of an existing information resource and therefore are relatively inexpensive. The appendix lists studies that have used administrative claims and records data for the six general purposes listed above. The studies are organized into four categories: diabetes; asthma; congestive heart failure (CHF), hypertension, and cardiovascular disease (CVD); and arthritis.

A common weakness of these types of analyses is their tendency to exclude plan members who are not continuously enrolled in the plan over a long time period. Noncontinuously enrolled members presumably are excluded from analysis because it is impossible for MCOs to identify costs or utilization during time periods when these patients were not enrolled in the plan. Typically, these studies examine health expenditures or determine the processes of care provided to patients, including patterns of medication prescribing. Because this information is not readily available for individuals who do not have insurance coverage for prescription drugs, these patients, too, are frequently excluded from analysis. Drug coverage is not an issue for Medicaid beneficiaries enrolled in MCOs, but it is common for Medicare beneficiaries to lack coverage in some parts of the country where Medicare payment rates for contracting MCOs are relatively low. Medicare MCOs are not required to offer prescription drug coverage. In the private sector, large employers typically offer prescription benefits, but coverage is much less common among smaller employers with low-wage workers.

These exclusions, although methodologically convenient, serve systematically to remove from analysis members of lower socioeconomic status and members with unstable employment situations, as it is these individuals who are both less likely to be continuously enrolled over long periods of time and less likely to have prescription drug coverage.

Benchmarking

From the perspective of the peer-reviewed literature, the most prevalent use of administrative claims and medical record data in chronic illness management is the comparison of care provided to practice guidelines or "best practice" benchmarks. MCOs compare their practices to externally developed guidelines, industry benchmarks, or practices at other MCOs. The classic example of this type of administrative and medical records data use is the National Committee for Quality Assurance (NCQA) accreditation and review process.

In the case of diabetes, MCOs frequently compare their performance to guidelines for care established by the American Diabetes Association (ADA). For example, Peters, Legorreta, Ossorio, and Davidson (1996) used administrative claims to identify the rate of retinal examinations and other recommended tests among diabetic enrollees in Health Net, an independent physician association (IPA)-network HMO in California. The study was initiated to satisfy HEDIS reporting requirements regarding retinal screening and was expanded to include other indicators of adherence to diabetic care guidelines. According to HEDIS guidelines for the retinal screening measure, the population was restricted to enrollees between the ages of 30 and 65.

Patients were identified through medical claims and pharmacy records. From a pool of 14,539 diabetics, a random sample of 384 patients was selected for medical record review (Peters et al., 1996).

Peters et al. (1996) found relatively low rates of adherence to ADA guidelines. Only 6% of patients received foot exams during their visits, and only 22% had been referred to an ophthalmologist for a retinal exam (Peters et al., 1996). Only 44% of patients had at least one HbA1c test during the year, and of those who did receive measurements, nearly 40% had values greater than 10.0 (well above the acceptable range for diabetic patients). As in most studies that identify study populations using administrative claims, the Peters et al. (1996) study required that patients be continuously enrolled for an extended period of time (24 months). It is not clear if patients were also required to have drug benefits to be included in the study. The results of this study support the common belief that diabetics in the United States do not receive care according to best-practice guidelines (Peters et al., 1996).

Martin, Selby, and Zhang (1995) used pharmacy claims to identify diabetic members of Kaiser Permanente of Northern California served by Kaiser's Oakland Medical Center. Medical chart review then was conducted to assess adherence to recommended guidelines for care and patient factors that affected this adherence. A primary purpose of this study was to examine the impact of race on adherence to diabetic care guidelines. Rates of adherence to various recommended procedures were slightly higher in the Martin et al. (1995) population than those reported by Peters et al. (1996), although the population exclusions in these two studies were different, and the populations are therefore not directly comparable. Martin et al. (1995) reported that between 53% to 65% of patients (depending on race) had evidence of annual retinal eye examination and about 60% of patients had documentation of an annual foot examination. The rate of at least one HbA1c test per year in the population ranged from 45% to 50% (Martin et al., 1995).

Identification of diabetic patients using pharmacy claims alone (as was done in the Martin et al., 1995, study) may fail to include a portion of the diabetic population, depending on the extent of pharmacy-benefit coverage in the population and the number of patients with non-insulin dependent diabetes mellitus (NIDDM) treated with diet alone. In the case of enrollees in Kaiser, the latter is more likely to be an issue than the former, as prescription-drug benefits are a standard part of most Kaiser plans. As with Peters et al. (1996), patients in the Martin et al. (1995) study were required to be continuous members of the Kaiser plan for 24 months prior to the window of time during which medical records were reviewed. Neither Martin et al. (1995) nor Peters et al. (1996) reported how many identified diabetics were eliminated from the analysis because of continuous enrollment requirements.

Jatulis et al. (1998) and Legorreta et al. (1998) reported adherence to National Asthma Education Project (NAEP) guidelines regarding anti-inflammatory and bronchodilator use among asthmatic patients in the Health Net system in California. For these studies, the authors used pharmacy records to identify asthmatic patients from among enrollees older than the age of 14 who were continuously enrolled for 12 months in 1995. These patients were targeted for a Health Survey for Asthma Patients. Patient data were collected both from survey responses and from pharmacy records. Thus, the sample was limited to those patients who responded to the asthma survey.

As reported in the case of diabetes care, adherence to care guidelines among asthmatic patients in the Health Net system was low (Jatulis et al., 1998; Legorreta et al., 1998). A significant proportion of patients used bronchiodilators as the first line of therapy, without maintenance anti-inflammatories (Jatulis et al., 1998). Although 72% of patients with severe asthma possessed anti-inflammatory inhalers, only 54% used these medications daily (Legorreta et al., 1998). Like other studies that use administrative claims to identify patient populations, this study faces possible limitations due to survey response bias; the studies of asthma care in the Health Net system are also limited by their continuous enrollment requirements. Although the studies of diabetes and asthma care described above report low levels of adherence to care guidelines for these conditions, they are likely to portray levels of adherence that are better than would be reported for the entire population with these conditions.

Assessment of Quality of Care

Closely related to the comparison to external standards is the use of administrative claims and medical records data to characterize the quality of chronic illness management practices within the MCO. For example, Marshall et al. (1996) reported the quality of care provided to diabetic Medicare beneficiaries enrolled in five Medicare managed care plans in Arizona. This study was conducted on behalf of Health Services Advisory Group, Inc., Arizona's peer-review organization. Medical records for 150 patients from each of the five plans were reviewed, using a checklist of quality indicators that included 10 services (e.g., retinal examinations, diabetes education, frequency of HbA1c testing) and 10 measures of patient status (e.g., existence of retinopathy, HbA1c levels, hospitalization rates) (Marshall et al., 1996).

Marshall et al. (1996) found that few of the standards of care for diabetic patients were met by the MCOs. About 29% of patients received between 1 and 4 of the recommended 10 services, 39% received 5 to 6 of the services, and only 32% received between 7 and 10 of the services. The Marshall et al. (1996) study did not focus on comparing the performance of the five plans to each other. Rather, results were reported in the aggregate. The authors suggested that the results of their analysis were intended primarily to provide baseline information for the plans to use to improve the quality of the care they delivered to diabetic patients. The authors pointed out that, because the same number of patient charts were reviewed for each plan, the results may underrepresent large plans and overrepresent smaller plans.

Alexander et al. (1999) examined both outpatient claims data and medical records to establish the degree to which blood pressure was controlled in a population of known hypertensives in Kaiser Permanente of Northern California. They note that "provider organizations generally do not know how well blood pressure is controlled in their populations, and there is no established method for obtaining this information" (p. 2073). Alexander et al. (1999) found that their estimate of control was sensitive to the standards they used. For example, control was substantially lower (at 14%) when it was based on achieving blood-pressure readings below established criteria on 75% or more of patient visits. Using any of three other measures (mean blood pressure across all visits, last recorded blood pressure, or readings below criteria on 50% or more visits), control was achieved for about 30% of known hypertensives. The authors observe that assessment of the implications of their findings is difficult, lacking prediagnosis blood-pressure levels and comparable data from other MCOs.

Gottlieb and Salem-Schatz (1994) used automated medical records to examine the quality of anticoagulation management among atrial fibrillation patients enrolled in Harvard Community Health Plan, then a staff-model HMO with 11 health care centers in Boston, Massachusetts. The authors used medical records to identify complication rates and patient characteristics. Rates of adverse events and patient bleeding times were compared to results of anticoagulation therapy that have been reported in clinical trials. Thus, this medical records study examined quality of care and also compared outcome measures to benchmarks reported in the clinical trials literature.

In general, the HMO patients included in the Gottlieb and Salem-Schatz (1994) study were more likely to have serious comorbidities, such as diabetes, than patients used in clinical trials. As a result, the authors reported that anticoagulation efforts among the HMO patients were slightly less successful at achieving target bleeding rates than clinical trials have been. The HMO patients also experienced more minor bleeding events than were reported for clinical trial patients. Stroke rates and major bleeding-event rates in the HMO population, however, were similar to those reported among clinical trial subjects (Gottlieb & Salem-Schatz, 1994).

Because of the necessarily continuous nature of anticoagulation therapy, the Gottlieb and Salem-Schatz (1994) study was not affected by requirements for continuous enrollment in the health plan. Patients whose anticoagulation therapy was shorter than 3 months in duration, or was interrupted for 1 month or more, were excluded from the study because of their less severe disease state.

Identification of Opportunities for Improvement

MCOs can take advantage of the fact that they have a defined population to construct organization-wide cost and utilization profiles using administrative claims and medical records data. These profiles then can be used to identify chronic illness management areas or cost centers that are in need of restructuring.

Using medical records data, Glauber and Brown (1994) determined the impact of cardiovascular disease on patient care costs and utilization among diabetic and nondiabetic patients enrolled in Kaiser Permanente's Northwest Region (Portland, Oregon). Patients were originally identified for the study population using hospitalization and pharmacy records and were required to have 3 years of continuous enrollment for inclusion. In addition, the authors noted that patients who had never been hospitalized for diabetes, who used diet alone to control their diabetes, or who filled prescriptions at nonsystem pharmacies were not identified as diabetic for the purposes of their study (Glauber & Brown, 1994).

The Glauber and Brown (1994) analysis identified a high-cost patient population for Kaiser Permanente's Northwest system: patients with both diabetes and cardiovascular disease. Still, the authors noted that, among these patients, more attention was paid to problems specific to diabetes, and less focus was placed on lipid management and other strategies to control the effects of CVD. Glauber and Brown (1994) recommended greater attention to cardiovascular risk factors among enrolled diabetic patients.

The identification of sources of costs among patients was also the focus of the Stempel, Hedblom, Durcanin-Robbins, and Sturm (1996) study of asthmatic patients enrolled in four United HealthCare plans. Asthmatic patients in this study were identified through pharmacy and medical claims and were required to have 6 months of continuous enrollment in the plan, somewhat mitigating the usual limitations caused by more lengthy continuous-enrollment requirements. In this study, the authors identified the sites of care where patient costs were the highest, as well as patient characteristics that were associated with higher costs. The authors found that patients who were younger and patients who were female had higher asthma expenditures overall. These two patient groups also were the least likely to use inhaled anti-inflammatories as maintenance medications. Based on these findings, Stempel et al. (1996) recommended increased early intervention among asthmatics, particularly among children and female patients.

The Stempel et al. (1996) and Glauber and Brown (1994) studies provide examples of how evaluative studies relying on administrative claims and medical records data are used by MCOs to identify potential areas for improvement in care.

Profiling of Clinics and Providers

Administrative claims are frequently used to profile practice patterns within clinics or relating to individual providers. The profiles indicate the level of adherence to practice guidelines at the provider, group, or clinic level and can be employed in initiating quality-improvement efforts. Other uses of profiling are to compare the practice style and outcomes of care delivered by specialists to that delivered by generalists, to construct bonus or incentive payments for physicians and to build provider networks that are outcomes based.

Several authors have addressed the limitations of individual-level provider profiling based on utilization data. In particular, Hofer et al. (1999) note that individual physician profiles explain little of the variation in utilization among patients. Profiling techniques that do not control for case mix (e.g., disease severity) and other patient factors (such as age, education, and income) can inaccurately attribute variation among patient groups to physician practice. Given the information traditionally available in administrative claims, it is difficult to adjust adequately for case mix and other patient factors, using this data source alone.

Even in a case of well-controlled case mix, Hofer et al. (1999) report that it is difficult to attribute variation among patients to individual physicians. Where variations in cost and utilization can be attributed to physician practice styles, the authors suggest that the true cost savings that could be achieved by eliminating physician effects are far less than generally estimated, once issues of reliability are taken into account (Hofer et al., 1999).

Because adequate case-mix adjustment is rare, the danger of individual physician profiling, according to Hofer et al. (1999), lies in the fact that discouraging more severely ill patients from visiting their practice would improve physicians' individual profiles. Hofer et al. (1999) have suggested that a better use of physician profiling would be to examine practice profiles by age cohort, care system, or geographic area.

The use of administrative claims by MCOs specifically for provider management is not generally reported in the peer-reviewed literature. Rather, more general profiles and comparisons of care across various classes of providers have been published. For example, Nyman, Hillson, Stoner, and DeVries (1997) used administrative claims to compare the extent of diagnostic testing used by allergists and nonallergists in caring for pediatric asthma patients enrolled in one United HealthCare plan. All patients with a diagnosis of pediatric asthma enrolled in the plan during 1992 were included in the study ($N = 1,574$). Information regarding the levels of diagnostic testing was compared to costs and outcomes of care for patients in the study population (Nyman et al., 1997). Nyman et al. (1997) attempted to adjust for case mix by controlling for sex, age, drug regimen, and new entrance into the plan.

Nyman et al. (1997) reported that, although allergists ordered more diagnostic tests than nonallergists for pediatric asthma patients, aggregate costs for patients treated by allergists were not higher than aggregate costs for patients treated by nonallergists. These results are unexpected because, in a nonrandomized setting, one would anticipate that specialists would treat more complex and consequently more costly patients. Study results also suggested a greater level of effectiveness in the care provided by allergists to asthmatic children (Nyman et al., 1997).

Westley et al. (1997) used retrospective review of medical records to examine the cost-effectiveness of an allergist consultation for asthmatic patients enrolled in Kaiser Permanente in Denver, Colorado. The medical records of 70 patients who had been referred to an allergist for a consultation and who had been enrolled in the Kaiser plan for a year prior to this referral were examined. Westley et al. (1997) reported that sick office visits, emergency room (ER) visits, and hospitalizations were all significantly less among patients in the time period after the allergist consultation as compared to the time period prior to the consultation. The authors concluded that, overall, referral to the allergist resulted in a cost savings of $2,100 per patient in the 12 months after the allergist consultation (Westley et al., 1997).

The cost savings reported in the Westley et al. (1997) study may not be generalizable to the entire asthmatic population of the MCO. Patients who attended the allergist consultation were identified for study retrospectively. Thus, there is no randomized control group of similar patients who were not seen by an allergist to which the results can be compared. The patients referred to the allergist may have been those most likely to benefit from the consultation. There is no evidence, therefore, that widespread referral of asthmatic patients within the MCO to an allergist would produce similar cost savings.

In both the Westley et al. (1997) and Nyman et al. (1997) studies, patients were only included in the study sample if they had been continuously enrolled for the specified study time period.

Characterization of High-Risk Patients

Through the identification and stratification of high-risk patients, administrative claims analysis and medical records review can be used as part of the care-improvement process itself. An initial step in the development of a systemwide disease management strategy might involve the identification and stratification of high-risk patients for future targeted interventions. In addition, patient characteristics and management practices that lead to adverse events can be identified using these data sources, in theory.

The characterization of high-risk patients by MCOs using administrative claims and medical records data has been most common for asthma. A typical example of this strategy is reported by Grana, Preston, McDermott, and Hanchak (1997). Using medical, pharmacy, and laboratory claims in combination with demographic data, Grana et al. (1997) risk-stratified asthmatic patients enrolled in U.S. Healthcare and built a model to predict which patients were at risk for hospital admissions. The goal of the modeling procedure was to identify patients who would most benefit from patient education and case management.

As is common in this type of predictive model building, Grana et al. (1997) used half of their eligible patient population as a model-building sample, and the other half as a validation sample to verify the accuracy of the model. Grana et al. (1997) selected the validation and model-building samples from two different years of data, to assure that the model was accurate across time periods. The authors' model was able to predict hospital admissions in the validation sample reasonably well, although it slightly overestimated hospitalization rates on a consistent basis.

Grana et al. (1997) also risk-stratified the patients in the sample based on hospital and ER use and reported that patients in the most severe risk category will receive more case management and education resources. It is unclear how these measures will be carried out specifically.

The danger of implementing a chronic illness management intervention targeted at specific MCO enrollees, based on the results of administrative claims analysis, is that patients may resist chronic illness management efforts if they are not directly the result of interactions with their own physicians. Increasingly, patients are becoming aware of the use of administrative and medical records data for cost management purposes. Strategies such as those proposed by Grana et al. (1997), which use administrative data to target individual patients for increased intervention, may be perceived by patients as a threat to their privacy. For example, according to a recent article in *Consumer Reports* ("Who Knows," 2000), several pharmaceutical companies conducted direct-mail promotions with patients whose names and addresses were culled from the pharmacy databases of Giant and CVS pharmacies. In one case, patients who had filled prescriptions for nicotine-replacement therapies were solicited regarding the use of Zyban in their efforts to quit smoking. According to *Consumer Reports* ("Who Knows," 2000), "the promotions stopped after the public complained" (p. 25).

In a patient-severity profiling study very different from Grana et al. (1997), Donahue et al. (1997) explored the ability of automated medical records to identify high-risk asthmatic patients enrolled in the Harvard Community Health Plan. The authors investigated the degree to which various patient symptoms, health behaviors, intervals between prescription refills, and diagnostic testing were accurately reported in the medical records. They concluded that the automated medical records used by the health plan did not provide sufficient information to assess disease severity (Donahue et al., 1997). The authors suggested that the current medical record format and information-collection process should be improved so that the automated medical record system used by the health plan could become a tool for improving care delivery to the most severe asthmatics in the system (Donahue et al., 1997).

Simulation of Disease Management Interventions

Administrative claims and medical records are, on occasion, used to simulate cost-effectiveness or impact on health outcomes of existing or proposed chronic illness management interventions within MCOs. However, there are relatively few studies of this type reported in the literature. Simulation analysis creates an opportunity to test chronic illness management strategies that may not have been fully exploited by MCOs to date. As with physician profiling, it is possible that MCOs are using this approach but have not published results in the peer-reviewed literature.

Lieu, Quesenberry, Sorel, Mendoza, and Leong (1998) developed a simulation model using administrative claims information for asthmatic children enrolled in 15 Kaiser Permanente of Northern California clinics. After building a predictive model that identified children at high risk for hospitalization, Lieu et al. (1998) simulated the cost-effectiveness of enrolling these children in a hypothetical asthma-education program. The intervention was compared to the usual care situation in which high-risk patients were not identified and no targeted disease management intervention was employed (Lieu et al., 1998).

In this type of simulation model, the impact of the intervention program is estimated by the authors based on previous use of the intervention in a (presumably) similar setting. In simulation modeling, the results depend critically on the defining assumptions. Assumptions used by Lieu et al. (1998) in their simulation related to the impact of the educational intervention on avoided hospitalizations, ER visits, medication changes, and nonacute outpatient visits. In addition, assumptions were made regarding the value and extent of work loss that would be prevented by the intervention.

Generally, authors of simulation models address the impact of model assumptions by providing a sensitivity analysis that explores how the results would change if model assumptions were altered. Lieu et al. (1998) included sensitivity analyses of several of their model parameters, presenting cost-effectiveness results in terms of cost savings for a range of values for assumed parameters.

In the end, Lieu et al. (1998) reported that their simulated intervention was not cost-effective, as it resulted in net costs to both the health plan and society. The model results were highly sensitive to model assumptions, reacting specifically to changes in the cost of the intervention and valuations of parents' work time. The authors argued that, although generally not cost-saving, the intervention could still be a useful chronic illness management strategy for the health plan to adopt because of benefits that were not given monetary value in the model (e.g., improved day-to-day symptom management by patients, increased self-efficacy among patients).

Two features of the Lieu et al. (1998) study make it unusual in the field of administrative claims analyses. First, the authors did not exclude patients without drug benefits (about 20% of the population), although one of the study's primary variables of interest was medication use. Second, the authors did not exclude patients who were not continuously enrolled in the health plan, instead including all patients with active enrollment at a single, predetermined point in time. This study population contained a significant number of Medicaid enrollees, and the decision to include patients regardless of length of continuous enrollment allowed for maximal inclusion of members of this population. The authors reported that these two inclusion decisions were made to "test the effectiveness of the asthma prediction models under real circumstances" (Lieu et al., 1998, p. 1174).

Demers et al. (1997) developed a cost-effectiveness model that simulated various strategies for avoiding the long-term complications of NIDDM, as proposed by Fletcher Allen Health Care (Vermont and upstate New York) for its patient population. They simulated the cost-effectiveness of six specific management strategies among Fletcher's enrollees in a single county of Vermont: diabetes education, use of a "care passport" to track care, access to medical supplies for patients, a sick-day protocol, peer support groups, and formal implementation of care guidelines. The authors gathered baseline information at the county-level regarding the rates of diabetes, diabetic complications, service utilization, and costs in the population. Future diabetic complications and cost savings from the six intervention strategies described above were modeled based on assumptions regarding participation in the various strategies and the potential impact of these strategies.

The authors simulated the impact of the interventions over a 15-year period. After 15 years, the authors estimated that, including the cost of the interventions themselves, use of the chronic illness management strategies would result in a $112.4 million cost savings due to reduced diabetic complications.

As in Lieu et al. (1998), the validity of the Demers et al. (1997) simulation results is conditional on the model assumptions. Assumptions regarding patient participation in disease management and the ability of each of the management strategies to reduce diabetic complications are not well-described in the article, nor is there definitive evidence in the literature that these particular intervention strategies would necessarily lead to substantial cost savings. Demers et al. (1997) did not report results of any sensitivity analyses testing the response of their model projections to changes in assumptions.

Summary

The six general uses of administrative claims and medical record review discussed in this chapter are not mutually exclusive. In fact, most studies using these data sources addressed more than one of the goals described above. As represented in the appendix, the majority of published studies using these data sources have occurred in the arena of diabetes and asthma management.

There are several advantages to the use of administrative claims and medical records data in the analysis of chronic illness management practices. These data sources already exist and are relatively inexpensive to access. Also, the use of administrative databases, in particular, provides investigators with large numbers of observations for analysis. Thus, in large MCOs, the occurrence and implications of rare complications can be investigated. In addition, investigators can split their study populations into model-building and validation groups.

There are several cautions that apply to studies using administrative claims and medical records data, however.

1. Identified samples frequently suffer from sample-selection bias, as individuals without drug benefits or who are not continuously enrolled over long periods of time are frequently excluded from the study population. As discussed above, this tends to systematically exclude enrollees with particular characteristics.
2. The criteria for identifying patients for inclusion may not accurately capture all enrollees with a particular condition. For example, identification of diabetics using pharmacy records alone will eliminate patients with conditions controlled by diet

alone from the study group. Similarly, diagnostic codes often are assigned to patients when a test is performed to rule out a particular condition. If care is not taken to identify codes associated with rule-out procedures, individuals may be erroneously identified as having a condition.
3. Although stratification by disease severity is often the goal of administrative claims studies, it is sometimes difficult to identify patient severity of illness using these data alone. For example, many studies of diabetic patients cannot distinguish between insulin-dependent diabetes mellitus (IDDM) and NIDDM patients. Recommended care guidelines for the two patient groups are substantially different, however.
4. Used alone, administrative claims cannot provide information regarding patient race and other sociodemographic variables.

The use of medical records data in research suffers from additional limitations:

1. Medical record abstraction is time consuming and labor-intensive and, therefore, expensive. Studies that use medical records as a data source tend to have smaller sample sizes than administrative claims studies.
2. Medical record keeping is subject to inconsistencies in data recording and frequent failure to record various important events such as the provision of patient education, exercise counseling, or smoking cessation advice. Medical records also are notorious for poor recording of medication dosage changes.

Finally, both administrative claims and medical records are limited by their inability to capture information on noncovered services sought by patients or services sought out of network.

Of the six potential uses of administrative claims and medical record review described above, the most limited in number of publications is the simulation of the cost of disease management interventions. If used properly, chronic illness management simulations can be a powerful tool for MCOs to identify their options for improving care to their chronically ill patients. One of the most challenging aspects of creating useful chronic illness management intervention simulation models is to adequately identify the impact that specific components of chronic illness management interventions will have on patient outcomes.

Of the different uses of administrative claims and medical records data, the identification of individual patients for targeted interventions has the greatest potential to generate controversy. As patients become more sensitive to the ways in which medical records information is used, MCOs may face increasing resistance to the use of this information to identify individual patients for intervention.

APPENDIX: Studies That Use Administrative Claims and Medical Records Review to Assess the Management of Chronic Illnesses in Managed Care Organizations

Goal of Analysis	Specific Focus	Reference	Data Used	Setting/ Data Source
Diabetes				
Benchmarking	Patient and plan features that are predictors of adherence to annual HbA1c and retinal screening guidelines	Bhattacharyya (1997)	Administrative claims	Hawaii Medical Service Association, private business claims file
	Adherence to American Diabetes Association (ADA) guidelines	Peters et al. (1996)	Administrative claims and medical record review	Health Net, an IPA-network HMO with contracting physicians throughout California
	Adherence to ADA guidelines	Martin et al. (1995)	Medical record review	Kaiser Permanente, Northern California (Oakland Medical Center)

Goal of Analysis	Specific Focus	Reference	Data Used	Setting/ Data Source
Assessment of quality of care	Quality of care delivered to diabetic Medicare patients	Marshall et al. (1996)	Medical record review	Consortium of five Medicare managed care plans in Arizona
	Development of a diabetes surveillance system	Engelgau et al. (1998)	Administrative claims	Three sites: Group Health of Puget Sound, Lovelace Health System, and one United HealthCare affiliate
Identification of opportunities for improvement	Costs for patients with diabetes and hypertension compared to costs for patients with only one of these conditions	Amin et al. (1999)	Administrative claims	A hybrid IPA- and group-model HMO (not identified)
	Identification of factors that drive costs for diabetic patients	Bhattacharyya & Else (1999)	Administrative claims	Hawaii Medical Service Association, private business claims file
	Excess costs of care for patients with diabetes and the proportion of costs dedicated to treating diabetic complications	Selby et al. (1997)	Administrative claims	Kaiser Permanente, Northern California
	Service utilization	Glauber & Brown (1992, 1994)	Administrative claims and medical record review	Kaiser Permanente, Portland, Oregon

Goal of Analysis	Specific Focus	Reference	Data Used	Setting/Data Source
Characterization of high-risk patients	High-risk patients, predictors of adverse events	Bhattacharyya (1998)	Administrative claims	Sample of MCOs from the Hawaii Medical Service Association, private business file claims
Simulation of disease management intervention	Cost-effectiveness of disease management for patients with NIDDM	Demers et al. (1997)		Fletcher Allen Health Care, an integrated delivery system in Vermont and upstate New York
Asthma				
Benchmarking	Adherence to National Asthma Education Project (NAEP) guidelines	Jatulis et al. (1998) Legorreta et al. (1998)	Administrative claims and patient survey	Health Net, an IPA-network HMO with contracting physicians throughout California
	Adherence to NAEP guidelines	Nestor et al. (1998)	Pharmacy and medical record review	Florida MCO (not identified)
	Health plan performance based on asthma hospitalizations	Jordan et al. (1995)	Medical record review and administrative claims	15 managed care plans and Medicaid managed care plans in Massachusetts
Identification of opportunities for improvement	Service costs and utilization	Lanes et al. (1996)	Pharmacy and medical records	Fallon Community Health Plan (central Massachusetts)
	Disease prevalence, cost centers	Stempel et al. (1996)	Administrative claims	Four of United Health Care's plans
	Hospital utilization	Osborne et al. (1996)	Medical record review	Kaiser Permanente, Northwest

Goal of Analysis	Specific Focus	Reference	Data Used	Setting/Data Source
Profiling of clinics and providers	Practice styles among specialists and generalists	Nyman et al. (1997)	Administrative claims	United Health Care plan located in the Northeast
	Cost-effectiveness of allergist consults	Westley et al. (1997)	Medical record review	Kaiser Permanente, Denver
Characterization of high-risk patients	Prevalence of chronic airflow obstruction, characterization of hospitalization and emergency-room use	Vollmer et al. (1998)	Administrative claims and hospital discharge records	Kaiser Permanente, Northwest Region
	Patient and practice features that predict hospitalization and emergency-room visits	Legorreta et al. (1998)	Administrative claims and patient survey	Health Net, an IPA-network HMO with contracting physicians throughout California
	Management practices that predict hospitalization and emergency-room visits	Lieu et al. (1997)	Pharmacy claims, medical record review, and phone interview	Kaiser Permanente, Northern California
	Identification and severity stratification of high-risk patients	Grana et al. (1997)	Administrative claims	Multiple U.S. Healthcare plans
	Identification and characterization of severe cases among adults	Donahue et al. (1997)	Pharmacy claims and medical record review	Harvard Community Health Plan
	20-year trends in hospitalization use by patients of all ages	Vollmer et al. (1992) Vollmer et al. (1993)	Administrative claims and hospital discharge records	Kaiser Permanente, Northwest Region

Goal of Analysis	Specific Focus	Reference	Data Used	Setting/Data Source
Simulation of disease management intervention	Simulation of cost-effectiveness of an asthma management program for children	Lieu et al. (1998)	Pharmacy records and administrative claims	15 Kaiser Permanente, Northern California, clinics
Congestive Heart Failure and Other Cardiovascular Illnesses				
Benchmarking	Adherence to National Cholesterol Education Project (NCEP) lipid-testing guidelines	Davis et al. (1998)	Administrative claims and medical record review	Two Prudential Health Care plan sites
Assessment of quality of care	Assessment of excessive anticoagulation	Lousberg et al. (1998)	Laboratory data and medical record review	Kaiser Permanente, Colorado
	Assessment of excessive anticoagulation	Gottlieb & Salem-Schatz (1994)	Pharmacy records and medical record review	Harvard Community Health Plan
	Assessment of hypertension control	Alexander et al. (1999)	Administrative claims and medical record review	Kaiser Permanente, Northern California
Arthritis				
Identification of opportunities for improvement	Predicting health care costs among osteoarthritis patients older than 60 years of age	Cronan et al. (1995)	Medical record review and patient survey	HMO members in San Diego County, California (HMOs not identified)
	Costs and utilization of health services for osteoarthritis and rheumatoid arthritis patients in a group model HMO	Lanes et al. (1997)	Administrative claims	Fallon Community Health Plan, central Massachusetts

References

Alexander, M., Tekawa, I., Hunketer, E., Fireman, B., Rowell, R., Selby, J., Massie, B., & Cooper, W. (1999). Evaluating hypertension control in a managed care setting. *Archives of Internal Medicine, 159,* 2673-2677.

Amin, S. P., Mullins, C. D., Duncan, B. S., & Blandford, L. (1999). Direct health care costs for treatment of diabetes mellitus and hypertension in an IPA-group-model HMO. *American Journal of Health System Pharmacy, 56*(15), 1515-1520.

Bhattacharyya, S. K. (1997). Monitoring patients with diabetes mellitus: An application of the probit model using managed care claims data. *American Journal of Managed Care, 3*(9), 1343-1350.

Bhattacharyya, S. K. (1998). Predicting hospitalization of patients with diabetes mellitus: An application of the Bayesian discriminant analysis. *Pharmacoeconomics, 13*(5), 519-529.

Bhattacharyya, S. K., & Else, B. A. (1999). Medical costs of managed care in patients with type 2 diabetes mellitus. *Clinical Therapeutics, 21*(12), 2131-2142.

Cronan, T. A., Shaw, W. S., Gallagher, R. A., & Weisman, M. (1995). Predicting health care use among older osteoarthritis patients in an HMO. *Arthritis Care and Research, 8*(2), 66-72.

Davis, K. C., Cogswell, M. E., Rothenberg, S. L., & Koplan, J. P. (1998). Lipid screening in a managed care population. *Public Health, 113*(4), 346-350.

Demers, D., Clark, N., Tolzmann, G., MacLean, C., Benedini, K., Farnham, P., Plant-DeHayes, A., & Nagy, P. (1997). Computer-simulated cost effectiveness of care management strategies on reduction of long-term sequelae in patients with non-insulin dependent diabetes mellitus. *Quality Management in Healthcare, 6*(1), 1-13.

Donahue, J. G., Weiss, S. T., Goetsch, M. A., Livingston, J. M., Greineder, D. K., & Platt, R. (1997). Assessment of asthma using automated and full-text medical records. *The Journal of Asthma, 34*(4), 273-281.

Engelgau, M. M., Geiss, L. S., Manninen, D. L., Orians, C. E., Wagner, E. H., Friedman, N. M., Hurley, J. S., Trinkaus, K. M., Shatin, D., & Van Vorst, K. A. (1998). Use of services by diabetes patients in managed care organizations: Development of a diabetes surveillance system. *Diabetes Care, 21*(12), 2062-2068.

Glauber, H., & Brown, J. (1992). Use of health maintenance organization databases to study pharmacy resource usage in diabetes mellitus. *Diabetes Care, 15*(7), 870-876.

Glauber, H., & Brown, J. (1994). Impact of cardiovascular disease on health care utilization in a defined diabetic population. *Journal of Clinical Epidemiology, 47*(10), 1133-1142.

Gottlieb, L. K., & Salem-Schatz, S. (1994). Anticoagulation in atrial fibrillation: Does efficacy in clinical trials translate into effectiveness in practice? *Archives of Internal Medicine, 154*(17), 1945-1953.

Grana, J., Preston, S., McDermott, P. D., & Hanchak, N. A. (1997). The use of administrative data to risk-stratify asthmatic patients. *American Journal of Medical Quality, 12*(2), 113-119.

Hofer, T. P., Hayward, R. A., Greenfield, S., Wagner, E. H., Kaplan, S. H., & Manning, W. G. (1999). The unreliability of individual physician "report cards" for assessing the costs and quality of care of a chronic disease. *Journal of the American Medical Association, 281,* 2098-2105.

Jatulis, D. E., Meng, Y. Y., Elashoff, R. M., Schocket, A. L., Evans, R. M., Hasan, A. G., & Legorreta, A. P. (1998). Preventive pharmacologic therapy among asthmatics: Five years after publication of guidelines. *Annals of Allergy, Asthma, & Immunology, 81*(1), 82-88.

Jordan, H. S., Straus, J. H., & Bailit, M. H. (1995). Reporting and using health plan performance information in Massachusetts. *The Joint Commission Journal on Quality Improvement, 21*(4), 167-177.

Lanes, S. F., Birmann, B. M., Walker, A. M., Sheffer, A. L., Rosiello, R. A., Lewis, B. E., & Dreyer, N. A. (1996). Characterisation of asthma management in the Fallon Community Health Plan from 1988 to 1991. *Pharmacoeconomics, 10*(4), 378-385.

Lanes, S. F., Lanza, L. L., Radensky, P. W., Yood, R. A., Meenan, R. F., Walker, A. M., & Dreyer, N. A. (1997). Resource utilization and cost of care for rheumatoid arthritis and osteoarthritis in a managed care setting: The importance of drug and surgery costs. *Arthritis and Rheumatism, 40*(8), 1475-1481.

Legorreta, A. P., Christian-Herman, J., O'Connor, R. D., Hasan, M. M., Evans, R., & Leung, K. M. (1998). Compliance with national asthma management guidelines and specialty care: A health maintenance organization experience. *Archives of Internal Medicine, 158*(5), 457-464.

Lieu, T. A., Quesenberry, C. P., Capra, A. M., Sorel, M. E., Martin, K. E., & Mendoza, G. R. (1997). Outpatient management practices associated with reduced risk of pediatric asthma hospitalization and emergency department visits. *Pediatrics, 100*(3), 334-341.

Lieu, T. A., Quesenberry, C. P., Sorel, M. E., Mendoza, G. R., & Leong, A. B. (1998). Computer-based models to identify high-risk children with asthma. *American Journal of Respiratory and Critical Care Medicine, 157*(4, Part 1), 1173-1180.

Lousberg, T. R., Witt, D. M., Beall, D. G., Carter, B. L., & Malone, D. C. (1998). Evaluation of excessive anticoagulation in a group model health maintenance organization. *Archives of Internal Medicine, 158*(5), 528-534.

Marshall, C. L., Bluestein, M., Chapin, C., Davis, T., Gersten, J., Harris, C., Hodgin, A., Larsen, W., Rigberg, H., Krishnaswami, V., & Darling, B. (1996). Outpatient management of diabetes mellitus in five Arizona Medicare managed care plans. *American Journal of Medical Quality, 11*(2), 87-93.

Martin, T. L., Selby, J. V., & Zhang, D. (1995). Physician and patient prevention practices in NIDDM in a large urban managed-care organization. *Diabetes Care, 18*(8), 1124-1132.

Nestor, A., Calhoun, A. C., Dickson, M., & Kalik, C. A. (1998). Cross-sectional analysis of the relationship between national guideline recommended asthma drug therapy and emergency/hospital use within a managed care population. *Annals of Allergy, Asthma, & Immunology, 81*(4), 327-330.

Nyman, J. A., Hillson, S., Stoner, T., & DeVries, A. (1997). Do specialists order too many tests? The case of allergists and pediatric asthma. *Annals of Allergy, Asthma, & Immunology, 79*(6), 496-502.

Osborne, M. L., Vollmer, W. M., & Buist, A. S. (1996). Periodicity of asthma, emphysema, and chronic bronchitis in a northwest health maintenance organization. *Chest, 110*(6), 1458-1462.

Peters, A. L., Legorreta, A. P., Ossorio, R. C., & Davidson, M. B. (1996). Quality of outpatient care provided to diabetic patients: A health maintenance organization experience. *Diabetes Care, 19*(6), 601-606.

Selby, J. V., Ray, G. T., Zhang, D., & Colby, C. J. (1997). Excess costs of medical care for patients with diabetes in a managed care population. *Diabetes Care, 20*(9), 1396-1402.

Stempel, D. A., Hedblom, E. C., Durcanin-Robbins, J. F., & Sturm, L. L. (1996). Use of a pharmacy and medical claims database to document cost centers for 1993 annual asthma expenditures. *Archives of Family Medicine, 5*(1), 36-40.

Vollmer, W. M., Buist, A. S., & Osborne, M. L. (1992). Twenty-year trends in hospital discharges for asthma among members of a health maintenance organization. *Journal of Clinical Epidemiology, 45*(9), 999-1006.

Vollmer, W. M., Osborne, M. L., & Buist, A. S. (1993). Temporal trends in hospital-based episodes of asthma care in a health maintenance organization. *The American Review of Respiratory Disease, 147*(2), 347-353.

Vollmer, W. M., Osborne, M. L., & Buist, A. S. (1998). 20-year trends in the prevalence of asthma and chronic airflow obstruction in an HMO. *American Journal of Respiratory and Critical Care Medicine, 157*(4, Part 1), 1079-1084.

Westley, C. R., Spiecher, B., Starr, L., Simons, P., Sanders, B., Marsh, W., Comer, C., & Harvey, R. (1997). Cost effectiveness of an allergy consultation in the management of asthma. *Allergy and Asthma Proceedings, 18*(1), 15-18.

Who knows your medical secrets? (2000, August). *Consumer Reports,* pp. 22-26.

6 The Effectiveness of Targeted Initiatives in Treating Chronic Illnesses

What is the evidence that specific programs implemented in managed care settings are effective in treating chronic illness? This begs the question: effective compared to what? The obvious answer is effective compared to care delivered in non-managed care settings. Because we define managed care as care organized around a defined population, it is difficult to compare the effectiveness to usual care, where there typically is not a defined population that can be used for comparison.

As an alternative approach, one could compare care delivered in managed care settings to treatment known to be desirable based on randomized, controlled studies. HEDIS measures suggest that managed care organizations (MCOs) do not perform as well as randomized, controlled efficacy trials, but this is understandable because randomized trials eliminate many of the confounding factors that make up the everyday care-delivery environment. Trials enroll volunteers, a group known to benefit more than nonvolunteers from placebos as well as effective interventions. In addition, randomized controlled trials dedicate significant resources to ensure compliance and follow-up, probably more than could be expected in real-world practice settings.

Outside of randomized controlled trials, in both non-managed care settings and managed care settings, it is clear that many actions known to be effective in improving (or at least monitoring) health status among the chronically ill are frequently not taken to the fullest extent (Wagner, 1997; Wagner, Austin, & Von Korff, 1996). For example, the Diabetes Control and Complications Trial (DCCT) demonstrated that the maintenance of near-normal blood glucose levels in diabetic patients can significantly reduce the occurrence of complications from diabetes, and the American Diabetes Association recommends that blood-glucose tests be conducted at least twice per year. Yet, few practice settings can boast adequate rates of HbA1c testing for the majority of their diabetic patients. Similarly, although these measures are also recommended by the American Diabetes Association, a relatively low percentage of diabetic patients receive annual dilated retinal exams, annual lipid testing, or regular foot examinations (Martin, Selby, & Zhang, 1995; Peters, Legorreta, Ossorio, & Davidson, 1996).

Several studies conducted in a variety of different practice settings, including MCOs, provide evidence that care for people with chronic illnesses typically falls short of desired goals. For example, Rubin, Dietrich, and Hawk (1998) reported that only 34% of diabetic patients had received an HbA1c test in the year prior to the implementation of Diabetes Net Care in seven HMO sites nationwide, which serve more than 7,000 diabetic patients. Similarly, only 23% of patients had received annual retinal eye exams, only 39% had received annual lipid screening, and only 2% had received foot exams (Rubin et al., 1998). Chicoye, Roethel, Hatch, and Wesolowski (1998) reported that, prior to a diabetes management intervention developed by Prime Care (a network model HMO in Wisconsin), only 44% of diabetic patients received annual HbA1c tests, and only 26% received annual eye exams. Prior to the development of the Episodes of Care program for diabetes management at Lovelace Health System, only 47.3% of diabetic patients received annual eye examinations (Friedman, Gleeson, Kent, Foris, & Rodriguez, 1998). At Health Net, a network HMO in California, only 20.9% of the eligible diabetic population received a retinal examination in the year preceding implementation of a diabetes management intervention (Legorreta, Hasan, Peters, Pelletier, & Leung, 1997).

Although they are recommended as the first line of therapy for both symptomatic and nonsymptomatic patients and are known to slow the progression of disease, ACE inhibitors are not prescribed to congestive heart failure (CHF) patients with recommended frequency. For example, among CHF patients released from Jewish Hospital at Washington University Medical Center, Rich et al. (1995; Rich, Gray, Beckham, Wittenberg, & Luther, 1996) found a baseline rate of ACE-inhibitor use of about 58%. Similarly, among asthma patients, the use rate of inhaled corticosteroids for asthmatics is low, despite clear recommendations for the use of inhaled corticosteriods as maintenance medications for both adult and child asthmatics. Buchner et al. (1998) reported that, in the year prior to implementation of an asthma management intervention in an independent physician association (IPA)-model HMO, only one in four asthmatic members had at least one pharmacy claim for inhaled corticosteriods. Still fewer asthmatic patients are educated in the use of metered dose inhalers (MDIs) and peak-flow meters (PFMs), devices that are argued to be useful in helping patients avoid the symptoms of asthma and acute asthma attacks (Boggs, Hayati, Washburne, & Wheeler, 1999).

Thus, in the area of chronic illness management in MCOs, there appears to be considerable room for improvement. Part of the appeal of MCOs is that they serve defined populations and therefore should be uniquely positioned to offer memberwide chronic illness management to their patients. However, even where MCOs have the structural and systemic mechanisms in place to improve the health of the chronically ill on a population-wide scale, the existence of these mechanisms does not automatically lead to improved patient outcomes (Wagner, 1997). This chapter focuses on specific programs implemented by MCOs for patients with diabetes, CHF, asthma, cardiovascular disease (CVD: hypertension, dyslipidemia, and coronary artery disease), and arthritis (osteo and rheumatoid). Using the peer-reviewed literature published between January 1985 and December 1999, we evaluate evidence of effectiveness of specific managed care programs in treating chronic illness by asking, Did the study find that the intervention improved the health of a population with a specific chronic disease?

Some Definitions

In this chapter, we use *effective* to describe a program where there was a statistically significant improvement compared to the organization's own usual care prior to program implementation, or compared to usual care in a similar setting. There are two ways to demonstrate effectiveness.

1. Did the intervention achieve a change known from an efficacy study to improve morbidity or mortality? For example, did implementation of a disease management intervention increase the number of CHF patients treated with ACE inhibitors?
2. Was a direct change in outcome demonstrated? Generally, large collaborative multi-organization studies like the DCCT are required to gather enough patients to demonstrate a significant change in mortality or morbidity. The usual outcomes measured in single organization studies are hospitalization rates, emergency room (ER) visits, costs, satisfaction, and functional status.

For our evaluation of specific programs, we note the potential for selection bias (due to volunteer bias or exclusion of complex cases) and secular trend bias. We also note studies in which indicators of program impact (measures of utilization or satisfaction, for example) may have served as poor proxies for patient health-status outcomes.

We use the term *population* to refer to the potential pool of individuals with the chronic disease. We found a large number of articles describing the success of specific programs. Most of these articles do not describe the potential eligible candidates for the program but simply focus on the individuals who were treated under the program. What percentage of the eligible patients were referred to the program? Were these patients representative of all eligible patients? Did the success of the program measurably improve the health of the entire denominator of eligible patients? Incomplete reporting of the eligible denominator represents a limitation in most of the studies that we reviewed.

The study of a nutritional intervention for diabetic patients reported by Franz et al. (1995) provides on example of a program focus with no discussion of how the eligible denominator was affected. The study describes a program for diabetes in which primary-care providers referred patients to the program. What were the referral criteria? What percentage of eligible patients within primary care were enrolled in the program? Although the study was conducted in a managed care setting, it reported only on patients experiencing the program.

We classified patient denominators as follows:

> *Programwide:* The study reports only on the results of the patients within a specific program, not the potentially eligible patients with the specific disease.
>
> *Memberwide:* The study reports the impact on all members with a specific diagnosis enrolled in a given health plan. That is, all potentially eligible patients with a specific disease are included.
>
> *Community-wide:* The study reports the impact on all individuals with a specific diagnosis within a defined geographic area.

A study must be conducted at least at the memberwide level to conclude that it improved the health of a population with a specific chronic disease. A community-wide approach to disease management is seldom attempted by MCOs. Exceptions to this are the community-wide Baltimore Alliance for the Prevention and Control of Hypertension and Diabetes (described by Gerber & Stewart, 1998) and the Fresno Asthma Project (described by Wilson et al., 1998). Both of these community-wide interventions involved MCOs as critical partners and are included in our review of the literature.

Many of the disease management programs described in this chapter (particularly those for asthma and CHF) are targeted toward high-risk patients. An exclusive focus on high-risk patients can be a highly effective and efficient use of resources. Most of the studies describing these interventions are identified in our review as programwide. However, it is not just their focus on high-risk populations that leads us to identify these disease management studies as programwide. Rather, the programwide categorization is appropriate because these disease management programs, as best we can determine given their descriptions, only monitor patients specifically enrolled in the disease management intervention.

A disease management program focused on high-risk patients also could include monitoring of care processes and/or outcomes for the entire population of patients with the disease to identify patients who could benefit from the program. We rarely found this to be the case, however. An intermediate step might be to evaluate care processes and health outcomes among all high-risk patients who would be eligible for the intervention, including those patients who did not participate for some reason (exclusionary diagnosis, refusal to participate, inability to contact, etc.) Again, this did not appear to be the case in the studies we reviewed.

Criteria for Study Selection

Based on a definition of managed care as a set of techniques used to influence the delivery of health services to a defined population, we conducted key-word searches of Medline and Health Star (as described in Chapter 1) to identify appropriate literature published between January 1985 and December 1999. Many articles identified through this search strategy were not considered appropriate for the purposes of this chapter. Articles were excluded for the following reasons:

- Publication in a non-peer reviewed journal
- Publication in a foreign language journal or focus on an intervention occurring outside of the United States
- Focus on an intervention occurring in a Veterans' Administration setting
- Focus on one portion of chronic illness management (e.g., a diabetes intervention that is geared toward increasing the rate of foot self-inspection, with no regard to other aspects of diabetes management)
- Use of only administrative claims or medical record review as a form of disease management within an MCO, without direct changes in patient care (see Chapter 5 for a discussion of studies of this type)
- Focus solely on development of an educational tool (frequently the case in the asthma and arthritis literature)

We found several studies based in academic centers but did not review these studies unless they contained a clear population focus. The tertiary focus of the academic center studies that we did review makes it difficult to identify the impact of interventions on the potential eligible patients within a referral network. Similarly, the set of potential eligible patients is difficult to identify in the case of hospital-based studies. For the most part, hospital-based studies were excluded from our review, precisely because of the inability to identify the eligible patient denominator for these interventions. However, in the case of CHF and CVD management, hospital-based studies so dominate the field of existing disease management interventions that selected studies were noted in the review if they were widely cited and if the patient populations were likely to include enrollees in MCOs.

We found great diversity in the articles we considered for inclusion in this chapter. Many of the articles describe innovative programs without evaluation of outcomes. These articles help to illuminate the range of efforts on the part of MCOs to manage care for enrollees with chronic illnesses. We did not include them here in part because of their large number, but primarily because our focus is on evaluating what we know, based on research, regarding program effectiveness. Most of the articles that we do include in this chapter focus on a program, rather than a defined population. Table 6.1 illustrates the dominance of programwide studies in the literature and the small proportion of studies in each disease category employing memberwide denominators.

Overview of Review Process

Summaries of the selected peer-reviewed literature are provided in the appendixes, with accompanying descriptive text. In addition, a table describing the specific features of each disease management intervention is provided. Wagner (1996) presents a model of chronic disease management in managed care settings that includes the components he argues are necessary to improve health outcomes for patients with chronic illness: (a) the use of evidence-based practice guidelines for care, (b) practice redesign (realignment of provider-patients roles, changes in appointment structure, increased patient follow-up), (c) patient education (with special focus on self-management of disease and psychosocial support), (d) use of expert systems (provider education and decision support tools), and (e) increased information resources (patient registries, outcomes feedback, care planning).

Table 6.1 Literature Search Results

	Diabetes	Asthma[a]	CHF	CVD	Arthritis[a]	Total
Total number of articles identified	73	166	51	61	48	399
Articles passing criteria for inclusion in review	31	23	16	17	2	89
Articles that are descriptive only, no formal evaluation of outcomes conducted	10	10	7	5	0	32
Articles that include evaluation of outcomes	20	13	9	12	2	56
Programwide	14	14	13	9	2	52
Memberwide	15	8	3	6	0	32
Communitywide	1	1	0	1	0	3

a. The total numbers of articles identified for asthma and arthritis are large relative to the number of articles included in the literature review due to the large number of pilot studies oriented toward developing patient education tools.

Our categorization of chronic illness management interventions differs from Wagner's model, but we follow an organizational structure that, like Wagner's, focuses on chronic illness management interventions at all levels of an MCO's operations. In the literature review appendixes and the tables describing intervention characteristics (Tables 6.2 through 6.8), the literature is organized in terms of its attention to care at (a) the patient level, (b) the provider level, or (c) the system level. Most disease management programs described include intervention features at a combination of two if not all three levels.

Interventions at the patient level include those that are directed exclusively at patients and do not involve providers. Patient-level interventions encountered in the literature include patient education, automated patient reminders, computer-aided interfaces for patients, and patient-specific care plans.

Provider-level interventions are those geared directly toward providers in an effort to educate, aid decision making, and change behavior. Provider-level interventions encountered in the literature include provider education, physician profiling, automated reminders, the implementation of guidelines and care protocols, and computer interfaces for physicians.

System-level interventions, the broadest category of intervention features, refers to program features that involve the introduction of new strategies of disease management into the organization. System-level interventions noted in the literature include use of multidisciplinary teams, nurse case management, miniclinics or dedicated days, nurse-managed miniclinics, use of pharmacists as care providers, alternative approaches to on-site contact with patients, referral to specialists, carve-outs, special management of complex cases, use of vendor products, partnerships with public entities, continuous quality improvement (CQI), and use of quality assurance mechanisms.

Because they involve the entire organization, interventions involving partnerships with public entities, CQI initiatives, or quality-assurance mechanisms tend to be memberwide, affecting all enrollees in a plan with a given chronic condition. These interventions are distinguished by the fact that they are top-down management strategies that make changes in patient care by addressing the organizational design of care within the MCO.

Most patient-, physician-, and system-level interventions occur at the programwide level, involving only those patients actually enrolled in a specific chronic illness intervention. There does exist overlap in the classifications of interventions. That is, an intervention may contain heavy emphasis both on patient education (patient-level focus) as well as on improvements in the process of care delivery through the use of alternative methods of patient contact (system-level focus). In the appendixes, studies are listed according to what appeared to us to be the dominant focus of the intervention. In Tables 6.2 through 6.8, which describe the individual characteristics of each intervention, the intervention feature that served as the cornerstone of the chronic illness management program is indicated with a (•). Other features of each intervention are indicated with an (X).

Diabetes

Most interventions for diabetes management include patient education as a crucial component. The DCCT trial provided definitive evidence that the maintenance of near-normal blood-sugar levels can decrease the risk of diabetic complications (The DCCT Research Group, 1993; Lasker, 1993; Mazze, Bergenstal, & Ginsberg, 1995; McCulloch, Glasgow, Hampson, & Wagner, 1994). Providers have long recognized the importance of self-management of disease to the maintenance of diabetic control. It is argued that improved self-management can be achieved through patient education (Etzwiler, 1972; Mazzuca et al., 1986; Rosenstock, 1985). More recently, the role of patient empowerment as a specific end goal of education has been investigated (Anderson, 1995; Anderson et al., 1995). In the studies reviewed below, if education is not the primary focus of an MCO's intervention for diabetes management, it is a key component.

Closely related to the concept of patient education in diabetes is the concept of the multidisciplinary team for patient care. Several of the studies described here evaluate MCO programs involving patient education regarding nutrition, exercise, insulin dosing, stress, sick-day management and home blood-glucose monitoring by providing patients with a team of resources, including physicians, nutritionists, certified diabetic educators, and, in some cases, mental health providers, exercise physiologists, and social workers (Abourizk, O'Connor, Crabtree, & Schnatz, 1994; Davidson, 1997; Edelstein & Cesta, 1993; Geffner, 1992; Graff, Bensussen-Walls, Cody, & Williamson, 1995; O'Connor et al., 1996; Rubin et al., 1998; Solberg et al., 1997). Frequently, these multidisciplinary teams are coordinated or led by nurse specialists or case managers (Davidson, 1997; Edelstein & Cesta, 1993; Graff et al., 1995; Rubin et al., 1998). An increased role for pharmacists in diabetic education and patient care has also been part of some diabetes management initiatives undertaken by MCOs (Gerber, Liu, & McCombs, 1998).

Several MCOs provide multidisciplinary care to their diabetic patients in the form of miniclinics or "diabetic days," which offer one-stop shopping where diabetic patients can receive all of their care and education (Abourizk et al., 1994; Friedman, 1996; Geffner, 1992; Peters &

Davidson, 1998; Peters, Davidson, & Ossorio, 1995; Wagner, 1995). Again, these miniclinics or dedicated days are often managed by nurse specialists.

Memberwide Interventions for Diabetes Management in MCOs

Of the literature reviewed for diabetes, only the project IDEAL studies by O'Connor and colleagues can be classified as memberwide (O'Connor & Pronk, 1998; O'Connor et al., 1996; Solberg et al., 1997). Project IDEAL (Improving Care for Diabetes Through Empowerment, Active Collaboration, and Leadership), a CQI initiative at the memberwide level, was first pilot-tested in a staff-model HMO in Minneapolis, Minnesota (HealthPartners). O'Connor et al. (1996) reported the outcomes of this pilot study, in which the results of the IDEAL model implementation were compared to diabetes care in a control clinic in the HMO's system.

The CQI process first pilot-tested at the clinic level was designed cooperatively by Health Partners, the Centers for Disease Control, and the Minnesota Department of Health. The initiative involved a 13-stage model of diabetes management that included assessment of current care practices, identification of barriers to care, development of innovative care strategies, implementation of these strategies, and evaluation of results (O'Connor et al., 1996). The initiative also included development of protocols for patient care and education.

Results of the pilot-test indicated improvement in health outcomes for diabetics enrolled in the intervention clinic (O'Connor et al., 1996). In the evaluation of most diabetes management interventions, the primary health-outcome indicator is change in HbA1c levels in the intervention population. The HbA1c provides a measure of glycemic control over a 12- to 14-week period. Because of the connection between glycemic control and reduced complications, changes in the HbA1c provide a useful indicator of the ability of an intervention to effect meaningful change in health outcomes.

In the year following the intervention, rates of annual HbA1c testing improved equivalently in both clinics. However, 12 months after program implementation, HbA1c levels in the intervention population improved to a significantly greater degree than improvements in the control population, after controlling for baseline readings. In addition, the proportion of patients categorized as being in good, fair, or poor control reflected significantly better control among the intervention population following program implementation. The disparity in HbA1c levels between treatment and control clinics, which had been observed at 12 months postintervention, widened by 18 months postintervention. The average HbA1c after 18 months in the intervention clinic was 7.9%, compared to 8.8% in the control clinic (O'Connor et al., 1996).

In addition to HbA1c results, O'Connor et al. (1996) also reported limited results pertaining to costs and utilization. Mean annual outpatient visits rose from 7.40 to 8.96 visits per patient in the control clinic and from 7.86 to 9.08 visits per patient in the intervention clinic. A 29% increase in outpatient charges for diabetes occurred during the study's time frame in the control clinic, compared to a 27% increase in the intervention clinic. O'Connor et al. (1996) suggested that these findings provided evidence that the intervention allowed for more intense diabetes care without an increase in outpatient costs. However, the cost estimates were based on the set of outpatient diabetic services only and (apparently) did not reflect the costs of program implementation and maintenance.

The first pilot project of Project IDEAL allowed for refinement of the program preliminary to further testing. Pilot studies in three additional Health Partners clinics began in 1996, funded by Health Partners, the Minnesota Department of Health, and the Centers for Disease Control's Diabetes Control Programs. Solberg et al. (1997) reported limited results from these pilot studies, identifying initial organizational barriers to implementation and methods through which staff acceptance of the program was enhanced. A review of care processes in the pilot clinics revealed that clinicians were not providing adequate management to their diabetics and highlighted the need in each clinic for systemic change (Solberg et al., 1997).

A randomized controlled trial of Project IDEAL in 13 Health Partners clinics (six intervention and seven control clinics) was initiated in January 1997, but Health Partners had difficulty recruiting clinics for the trial. Several clinic directors felt that their staff was already overwhelmed with patient care. Other clinics were in the process of developing their own diabetes management programs or were taking part in trials of competing programs. Study results from the randomized controlled trial have not yet been published.

Diabetes Management Interventions in MCOs at the Programwide Level

Several MCOs have demonstrated an impact on health outcomes and processes of care among subsets of their diabetic enrollees through chronic illness management interventions that occur at the programwide level. In these interventions, not all eligible patients within the MCO are enrolled. Decreases in enrolled patients' HbA1c levels have been achieved in MCOs through nutrition therapy (Franz et al., 1995) and through nurse-specialist management of care (Aubert et al., 1998; Davidson, 1997; Peters et al., 1995).

Other health indicators, including body-weight changes, cholesterol and triglyceride levels, creatinine levels, and the frequency of adverse events, have been used to gauge the impact of programwide diabetes management interventions in MCOs. Aubert et al. (1998) measured (but did not detect) changes in cholesterol, triglyceride, and creatinine levels and changes in the frequency of adverse events among diabetic patients enrolled in a nurse-managed intervention in two clinics of the Jacksonville (Florida) Health Care Group. Franz et al. (1995) reported success in improving cholesterol levels, fasting blood-glucose levels, waist-to-hip ratio, and triglyceride levels with a nutritional therapy intervention for patients enrolled in three outpatient diabetes centers affiliated with MCOs.

Improvements in health status, as demonstrated by reductions in HbA1c levels, weight loss, changes in cholesterol and triglyceride levels, and other laboratory values provide a direct measure of the success of a diabetes-intervention program. Process improvements in care for diabetic patients provide other markers of the success of an intervention. The use of process improvements as an evaluative tool is common for diabetes management interventions because a set of easily measured processes have been defined by the American Diabetes Association as appropriate care. Although they are not a measure of improved health in a diabetic population, improvements in the processes of care for this population are assumed to be predictive of measurable improvements in health status. That is, population-wide reductions in

HbA1c levels are not likely to occur if fewer than 50% of the diabetic population receives an HbA1c test with recommended frequency. Likewise, decreases in diabetic retinopathy rates are not likely without consistent retinal screening in the diabetic population.

Because of HEDIS reporting requirements, frequency of HbA1c testing and rates of annual retinal eye examinations are the most common process indicators used to measure program success in MCOs. Other process indicators that have been used to evaluate interventions include foot-examination rates, lipid-panel testing rates, and rates of home blood-glucose monitoring among diabetics. Interventions in MCOs in which the primary goal is to improve the processes of care for diabetic patients are successful, in general. Systems of mailings and reminders to physicians and patients regarding the importance of retinal eye exams resulted in increased annual retinal examination rates in diabetic populations enrolled in Primecare in Wisconsin and Health Net in Woodland Hills, California (Chicoye et al., 1998; Legorreta et al., 1997). CQI interventions aimed at system-level changes in the management of diabetic populations, as implemented by Primecare of Wisconsin and Lovelace Health System of New Mexico, improved laboratory testing and retinal screening rates among diabetic enrollees (Chicoye et al., 1998; Friedman, 1996; Friedman et al., 1998).

As mentioned above, whereas demonstrations of improvements in the processes of care for diabetic patients are numerous, studies that demonstrate the connection between improvements in process and actual improvements in health outcomes are less common. Unlike process improvements in diabetes management, patient satisfaction with management strategies has not emerged as an indicator of program success in the peer-reviewed literature. This is surprising, given the high level of self-management of disease required for successful health outcomes in diabetes.

Interventions for Diabetes Management With Unknown Population Denominators

Our review of the literature includes several studies of diabetes management interventions that are likely to have included enrollees in MCOs but for which the eligible or target population is difficult to identify. These programs often are based in a hospital or an urban outpatient clinic affiliated with a hospital. They are briefly noted in this review because portions of their patient populations are likely to have been managed care enrollees. For example, McNabb, Quinn, Murphy, Thorp, and Cook (1994) studied the impact of the "In Control" program, an educational intervention for diabetic children. The children in the McNabb et al. (1994) study were all treated in the diabetes clinic of a large metropolitan children's hospital in Chicago, Illinois. In this study, enrollment in a 6-week educational program led to significant increases in the reported responsibility taken by children for their own care (McNabb et al., 1994). This increase in responsibility for self-management, however, was not linked to improved HbA1c levels in the patient group. The evaluation period for the study was short (12 weeks following initiation of a 6-week intervention) and may not have allowed sufficient time for changes in glycemic control to be captured by HbA1c levels. Because the intervention took place in a large teaching hospital, it is not clear from the study what proportion of the patients were managed care enrollees. Similarly, it is not clear how interventions described by McNabb et al. (1994), Smith et al. (1998), Abourizk et al. (1994), and Edelstein and Cesta (1993) are related to managed care or managed care settings.

Summary

Of the memberwide interventions for diabetes described in the literature, only O'Connor et al. (1996) provides formal evaluation results. An intervention that included an expanded role for nurses in the management of diabetic patients, described by Graff et al. (1995), and the Episodes of Care program developed by Lovelace Health System, as described by Friedman (1996), Friedman et al. (1998), and Terry (1997), also were implemented at the memberwide level. However, we did not find formal evaluations of these interventions in the peer-reviewed literature.

Overall, in the published literature, interventions that seek to improve the frequency of HbA1c testing and improve other processes of care for diabetic patients appear to be successful. Improvements in rates of HbA1c testing, lipid testing, and retinal screening are initial steps in improving patient outcomes in diabetes. Currently, the literature on diabetes management lacks formal evaluations of diabetes interventions in MCOs that link improvements in processes of care to improvements

(text continues on p. 131)

Table 6.2 Components of Diabetes Management Programs

Level of Focus	Characteristic	1	2	3	4	5	6	7	8	9	10	11	12	13	14	15	16	17	18	19	20	21	22	23	24	25	26	27	28
Patient	Patient education	•	•	•	•			X	X	X	X	X	X	X	X		X	X	X	X	X	X		X					X
	Automated patient reminders			X										X	X	X				X	X	X				X			
	Computer interface for patients—high level																												
	Patient-specific written management plan																												
Provider	Provider education			X		•							X			X				X							X	X	
	Physician profiling						•																X						
	Automated physician reminders																				X	X				X			
	Guidelines/protocols	X	X			X			•	•	X	X		X	X	X	X	X			X	X	X	X	X	X	X	X	X
	Computer interface for provider—high level						•			X					X	X				X		X		X				X	X
System	Multidisciplinary team			X				X	•			X				X						X		X	X	X	X	X	X
	Nurse case management								X	X	•	•	•	•	•	•				X								X	X

Level of Focus	Characteristic	Reference																										
		1	2	3	4	5	6	7	8	9	10	11	12	13	14	15	16	17	18	19	20	21	22	23	24	25	26	27	28
	Mini-clinic or dedicated day																					X	X					X	
	Nurse-managed mini-clinic												X				•												
	Pharmacist as care provider								X									•											
	Alternative approaches to on-site contact								X		X								X										X
	Nurse home-visits																												
System	Formal relationships with external resources			X															X		X								
	Referral to specialist																												
	Carve-outs							•																					
	Special management of complex cases																			X						X			X
	Vendor products																		•	•		X		•	X				
	Public/private partnership																		•		X					X	X		

(Continued)

Table 6.2 (Continued)

Level of Focus	Characteristic	Reference																												
		1	2	3	4	5	6	7	8	9	10	11	12	13	14	15	16	17	18	19	20	21	22	23	24	25	26	27	28
	Continuous quality improvement																				•	•	•	X		•	•	•	•
	Quality assurance																												

X = characteristic of program
• = most emphasized feature of program

1. Franz et al. (1995)
2. McNabb et al. (1993)
3. Singer (1995)
4. McNabb et al. (1994)
5. Benjamin et al. (1999)
6. Smith et al. (1998)
7. Abourizk et al. (1994)
8. Sadur et al. (1999)
9. Domurat (1999)
10. Aubert et al. (1998)
11. Edelstein et al. (1993)
12. Graff et al. (1995)
13. Peters et al. (1995)
14. Peters & Davidson (1998); Davidson (1997)
15. Legorreta et al. (1996)
16. Geffner (1992)
17. Gerber et al. (1998)
18. Gerber and Stewart (1998)
19. Rubin et al. (1998)
20. Chicoye et al. (1998)
21. Friedman et al. (1996, 1998); Terry (1997)
22. Gilmet et al. (1998)
23. Ginsberg et al. (1998); Mazze et al. (1994)
24. Heinen et al. (1993)
25. O'Connor et al. (1996); O'Connor & Pronk (1998)
26. Solberg et al. (1997)
27. Wagner (1995)
28. Joshi & Bernard (1999)

in patient outcomes. Also, as is the case throughout this chapter, it may be that this literature is subject to publication bias; that is, studies that have significant findings may be more likely to be submitted and accepted.

Many of the studies reviewed here share common limitations. First, several describe disease management interventions in detail but provide little in the way of formal evaluations of the impact of these programs. In addition, several of the programwide interventions suffer from small sample sizes, which hampers both their generalizability and their ability to detect significant changes in patient outcomes over time.

A more severe threat to generalizability is presented by volunteer or attrition bias in the study population. Franz et al. (1995) evaluated a nutritional intervention using a population that was recruited through public advertisements (Franz et al., 1995). McNabb et al. (1994) and Aubert et al. (1998) lost a significant portion of their patient populations when study recruits either refused to continue with the study or failed to attend their first appointments. In studies of this type, patients who volunteer or remain in the intervention may represent a more motivated patient group, who are then predisposed to better outcomes as a result of the intervention. In the examination of a nurse-managed diabetes program by Davidson (1997) and Peters and Davidson (1998), 34% of the intervention group was reported lost to follow-up because of a change in insurance status. This study could suffer from attrition bias due to the fact that populations with unstable insurance status tend to be younger, lower socioeconomic, minority populations. Additional methodological limitations relating to the reviewed studies are noted in Appendix A. Reviewed studies of diabetes interventions in managed care settings are presented in Appendix A; Table 6.2 details specific components of each intervention.

Asthma

Several accepted-practice standards exist for the care of asthma in children and adults. The second report of the Expert Panel of the National Asthma Education and Prevention (NAEP) Program (National Institutes of Health) reiterated the importance of both the use of inhaled anti-inflammatory agents and patient education as key components of asthma management for adults and children (NAEP Program, 1997). Inhaled anti-inflammatory medications (inhaled corticosteroids) used regularly, with inhaled beta-agonists for quick relief of sudden attacks, is the recognized first line of therapy for patients with mild to severe asthma (Homer, 1997; Lozano & Lieu, 1999; O'Brien, 1997; Self & Nolan, 1997; Sullivan et al., 1996).

Home monitoring with a PFM is recommended to provide an indication of the onset of attacks and for medication-dosage modification and is generally suggested for patients over the age of 6 (Homer, 1997; Lozano & Lieu, 1999; NAEP Program, 1997; O'Brien, 1997; Self & Nolan, 1997). Furthermore, the use of spacers and MDIs for medication delivery is recommended, particularly for children with asthma (O'Brien, 1997; Self & Nolan, 1997).

As in diabetes, self-management education is a crucial component of most asthma initiatives (Becker, McGhan, Dolovich, Proudlock, & Mitchell, 1994; Clark et al., 1981; Jones, Jones, & Katz, 1987a; Kotses et al., 1991; Maiman, Green, Gibson, & MacKenzie, 1979; NAEP Program, 1997; Self & Nolan, 1997; Sullivan et al., 1996). In asthma care, this education generally focuses on recognition of symptoms, management of acute attacks, the importance of maintenance medications, and the use of PFMs and MDIs. Self-management education has been demonstrated to decrease school absences and ER visits among children and adults (Clark et al., 1981; Greineder, Loane, & Parks, 1995, 1999; Lewis, Rachelefsky, Lewis, de la Sota, & Kaplan, 1984; Stevens & Weiss-Harrison, 1993), although results of studies of the direct impact of self-management education on days missed from school or work, ER use, and acute attacks are frequently mixed (Maiman et al., 1979; Sullivan et al., 1996). Sullivan et al. (1996) reported that asthma-education initiatives were most successful at improving outcomes when they were targeted at high-risk populations.

Recognition of the importance of education in the management of asthma has led to the development of a number of asthma-education programs, including Open Airways (Becker et al., 1994; Clark et al., 1981; Kaplan et al., 1986), Living With Asthma (Creer et al., 1988), The Family Asthma Program (Hindi-Alexander & Cropp, 1984), Wheezers Anonymous (Snyder, Winder, & Creer, 1987), Asthma Care Training (ACT) for Kids (Lewis et al., 1984, 1987; Lewis, Rachelefsky, Lewis,

Leake, & Richards, 1994), AIR WISE (Wilson-Pessano & McNabb, 1985), AIR POWER (Wilson-Pessano & McNabb, 1985), The Childhood Asthma Project (Hendricson et al., 1994, 1996) and You Can Control Asthma (Taggart, Zuckerman, Lucas, Acty-Lindsey, & Bellanti, 1987; Taggart et al., 1991). Primarily, these educational interventions have been developed for children, although some have been designed specifically for adults or later adapted for use with adults (Kowal, 1997; Snyder et al., 1987, Wilson et al., 1993; Wilson-Pessano et al., 1987). Several of these programs were developed specifically for inner-city, minority or Hispanic children (ACT for Kids, Open Airways, The Childhood Asthma Project). Peer-reviewed studies of the implementation of these education programs in MCOs are included in this literature review.

Memberwide Interventions for Asthma Management in MCOs

Only a study by Buchner et al. (1998) met our criteria of an intervention for a memberwide population of patients with asthma. Buchner et al. (1998) report the results of a chronic illness management program implemented in an IPA-network HMO (Mid-Atlantic Medical Services, Inc). The intervention used physician and patient education, with special focus on National Heart, Lung, and Blood Institute guidelines. Although this intervention likely increased drug costs as a result of increased compliance, it may be economically sustainable because of the decreased hospitalization rates that resulted.

The Buchner et al. (1998) study used a number of outcome measures, including patient knowledge indicators, quality-of-life, and satisfaction measures. Of greatest significance, however, were the improvements achieved by the initiative in processes of care and population health outcomes. The authors reported that, in the baseline year, one in four patients with asthma had one or more prescriptions for inhaled corticosteroids. This rate increased to one in three patients in the year following the intervention. Increases of a similar magnitude occurred in filled inhaled corticosteroid prescriptions among patients with prior hospitalizations and ER visits. The number of patients receiving chronic therapy (four or more prescriptions for inhaled corticosteroids within the year) increased by 25% overall (Buchner et al., 1998).

In terms of clinical outcomes, an 18% reduction in the number of patients hospitalized for asthma occurred in the follow-up year (from 5.6% to 4.6%, $p < .001$). Similarly, the authors observed a 39% reduction in the number of patients with multiple hospitalizations (from 0.84% to 0.51%, $p < .05$). The authors do not report the change (if any) in hospitalization rates for the IPA population as a whole, so it is difficult to determine if these decreases in hospitalization rates were an artifact of temporal trends or a result of the intervention. No change in the frequency of ER visits was noted following the intervention (Buchner et al., 1998).

The Buchner et al. (1998) study also reported changes in health-related quality of life (HRQOL), an outcome variable used relatively infrequently in the program evaluations we reviewed. Among adults, no changes in general well-being, using the SF-36, were reported in this study. However, there were improvements in quality of life (QoL) as measured by disease-specific scales (Buchner et al., 1998). Parents reporting HRQOL for their children indicated significant increases in both generic and disease-specific measures of QoL (Buchner et al., 1998).

Asthma Management Interventions in MCOs at the Programwide Level

Several asthma management interventions have been undertaken by MCOs at the programwide level (where not all eligible patients served by the MCO are targeted by the intervention). These initiatives have achieved improvements in health and process outcomes for asthmatic members to varying degrees.

Writing on behalf of the National Asthma Education and Prevention Program Working Group, Sullivan et al. (1996) recommended several outcome indicators for use in the evaluation of asthma disease management interventions, including (a) reported symptoms (such as reported acute events or number of sick days), (b) measures of lung function (such as forced expiratory volume or peak expiratory flow), (c) functional status and HRQOL, (d) indicators of behavior change (such as patient and family management behaviors), and (e) health services utilization (such as ER visits, hospitalizations, and acute care visits). In addition, evaluations of management interventions for asthma have included the assessment of educational outcomes (such as skill mastery and patient self-confidence), calculation of cost-effectiveness, and measurement of the adherence of physicians to medication-prescribing guidelines (e.g., the proportion of patients using inhaled anti-inflammatories). All of these outcome measures were used in various combinations in the evaluation of programwide asthma management interventions in MCOs.

By far the most commonly used indicators of program success were reductions in ER or acute care facility visits and hospitalizations. Several educational interventions used hospitalization and ER visit rates as their primary outcome variables of interest. Lewis et al. (1984) reported significant reductions in ER visits and borderline significant reductions in hospitalizations among intervention group children as compared to controls through the implementation of ACT for Kids in Kaiser Permanente of Los Angeles. In two separate studies, both focusing on an asthma outreach program for inner-city children enrolled in the Harvard Community Health Plan, Greineder et al. (1995, 1999) reported significant decreases in both ER visits and hospitalizations in the intervention population. However, in an adaptation of AIR WISE and AIR POWER for adults enrolled in Kaiser Permanente of Northern California, Wilson et al. (1993) noted no significant decrease in hospitalization events and mixed results in the area of ER and acute visit reductions.

Interventions without a primary focus on education also have achieved reductions in ER visits and hospitalizations. Zeiger et al. (1991) demonstrated a decrease in ER visits among intervention group patients enrolled in a Kaiser Permanente HMO in San Diego, California, who were randomly assigned to receive evaluation by an allergy specialist. Kropfelder (1996) reported significant decreases in both ER visits and hospitalizations following the implementation of a case management system in a Kaiser Permanente plan in Baltimore, Maryland. Decreases in acute care visits in this study were accompanied by a significant increase in routine outpatient visits among the enrolled population (Kropfelder, 1996).

Clinical measures of lung function, such as forced expiratory volume as measured by spirometry, are more frequently used in the clinical trial literature than in the evaluation of chronic illness management interventions. Patient and physician reports of asthma symptoms are typically used in the program-evaluation literature to determine the impact of asthma management programs on health outcomes. In their educational intervention for adult asthmatics enrolled in five Kaiser Permanente of Northern California plans, Wilson et al. (1993) observed no significant difference between intervention and control group patients in forced expiratory volume. However, the authors did observe significant improvements in "asthma bother ratings," symptom days, physician evaluation of symptoms, and physical activity management among intervention-group patients (Wilson et al., 1993). Following implementation of the Wee Wheezers educational program for parents of preschool-age children with asthma enrolled in the Aspen Medical Group (St. Paul, Minnesota), Wilson et al. (1996) observed a significant increase in symptom-free days among children in the intervention group as compared to controls. A significant decrease in parental sleep interruptions among parents of intervention-group children as compared to parents of controls also was observed.

Skill attainment, behavior change, and improved compliance are frequently measured in the assessment of educational interventions for asthma management in MCOs. The impact of educational interventions on long-term skill attainment and knowledge about asthma has been mixed. Lewis et al. (1984) noted no differences either pre- versus postintervention or between control and intervention groups in knowledge about asthma or self-ratings of health status among children enrolled in ACT for Kids in the Kaiser Permanente Sunset Clinic (Los Angeles, California). However, intervention-group patients demonstrated increased skill in managing asthma, increased responsibility in managing asthma, and increased family communication regarding asthma symptoms (Lewis et al., 1984). Wilson et al. (1993) observed improvements in patients' bedroom environments and improvements in MDI-use techniques among adults from five Kaiser Permanente of Northern California plans who were enrolled in AIR POWER and AIR WISE. Studies of educational interventions in MCOs also have used patient satisfaction with the educational program, patient attendance at educational sessions, and patient assessment of program utility as indicators of program success (Moe et al., 1992).

Costs have been used by MCOs to measure the success of program-wide asthma management interventions. Lewis et al. (1984) reported a decrease in costs of $180 per child per year enrolled in the ACT for Kids educational intervention in an MCO (in 1984 dollars). Greineder et al.

(1995) reported a cost savings of $11.67 for every $1 spent on an asthma outreach nurse for their asthma outreach program. Unfortunately, because of differences in calculation methods, these types of cost-effectiveness measures are often not comparable to one another.

Summary

Of several memberwide interventions included in our review (Goonan, Healy, Jordan, Zazzali, & Horowitz, 1993; Kowal, 1997; Plaut, Howell, Walsh, Pastor, & Jones, 1996; Stevens & Weiss-Harrison, 1993), only the Buchner et al. (1998) study presented a formal evaluation of the impact of the program on patient outcomes. Improvements in health outcomes in this study population were not dramatic. It may be difficult for MCOs to achieve improvements in health costs and outcomes with asthma management strategies that are restricted to the MCO's member population and its physical structure (i.e., clinics, hospitals, etc.) as the location of care management. Evidence from the literature would suggest that the successful chronic illness management programs for asthma are most often those that serve minority, low socioeconomic status, and inner-city patient populations. It is these populations in which asthma prevalence and severity are the greatest. The Fresno Asthma Project described by Wilson et al. (1998) represents a community-wide intervention that engaged MCO partners in asthma management outside of the traditional confines of the health care setting. Unfortunately, we found no published evaluation results for this project.

In addition, evidence from programwide interventions suggests that MCOs are most likely to achieve success in asthma management when they focus on their high-risk populations: those asthmatics with recent ER visits or hospitalizations. Of the literature reviewed, interventions described by Wilson-Pessano et al. (1987), Wilson et al. (1993), Forshee et al. (1998), Moe et al. (1992), McNabb, Wilson-Pessano, Hughes, and Scamagas (1985), Zeiger et al. (1991), Greineder et al. (1995, 1999), and Kropfelder (1996) enrolled only patients identified as high risk into asthma management intervention programs.

As in the literature reviewed for diabetes management programs, several of the studies reviewed for asthma contain common limitations. Many provide detailed descriptions of the asthma management intervention with limited information pertaining to the impact of the intervention on the patient population. Several studies suffer from threats to generalizability of findings due to volunteer or attrition bias. The generalizability of the results presented by Forshee et al. (1998) and Wilson et al. (1996) is limited by refusals to participate and losses to follow-up. Lewis et al. (1984) reported that those enrollees who dropped out of their program before completion were overwhelming Latino and African American.

Results of an education intervention for inner-city children in Chicago, as described by Griffin, McNabb, and Shields (1989) and Shields, Griffin, and McNabb (1990), are difficult to interpret because low program attendance significantly hampered the researchers' ability to deliver the disease management intervention as originally planned. This intervention may have failed because it was not designed to address the unique needs of a low income, inner-city, asthmatic population; namely, patients and their parents were unable to find the time, transportation, and child care needed to attend educational sessions at the clinic site. Literature reviewed relating to asthma management is presented in Appendix B; details of specific intervention characteristics are listed in Table 6.3.

Congestive Heart Failure

The management of CHF is of interest to MCOs, particularly those serving Medicare populations, because of the high prevalence and substantial treatment costs associated with the disease. CHF is a particularly pervasive problem among those older than age 65 and is the leading discharge diagnosis for hospitalized individuals in this age group (Abraham & Bristow, 1997; Wilkes, Dukes, Feagles, Leong, & Allen, 1999).

There exists a widely recognized set of evidence-based guidelines for CHF management, particularly in the area of pharmacotherapy (Abraham & Bristow, 1997; Institute for Clinical Systems Improvement [ICSI], 1998). ACE inhibitors are universally recommended as the first line of therapy for CHF patients with both systolic and diastolic

(text continues on p. 141)

Table 6.3 Components of Asthma Management Programs

Level of Focus	Characteristic	1	2	3	4	5	6	7	8	9	10	11	12	13	14	15	16	17	18	19	20	21
Patient	Patient education	•	•	•	•	•	•	•	•	X	X	X	X	X	X	X	X		X	X	X	X
	Automated patient reminders																		X			
	Computer interface for patients—high level																					
	Patient-specific written management plan				X										X							
Provider	Provider education	X								•	•										X	X
	Physician profiling																					
	Automated physician reminders																		X			
	Guidelines/protocols					X					X	X	X	X					X	X	X	X
	Computer interface for provider—high level																	X	X			
System	Multidisciplinary team	X									X					X		X	X			
	Nurse case management			X		X					X				•	X		X				
	Mini-clinic or dedicated day																		X			
	Nurse managed mini-clinic												•	•								
	Pharmacist as care provider																				X	
	Alternative approaches to on-site contact			X		X	X						X	X	X						X	

(Continued)

139

Table 6.3 (Continued)

Level of Focus	Characteristic	Reference																				
		1	2	3	4	5	6	7	8	9	10	11	12	13	14	15	16	17	18	19	20	21
System	Nurse home visits										X					•					X	X
	Formal relationships with external resources									X											X	
	Referral to specialist	X										•					•					
	Carve-outs																					
	Special management of complex cases	X		X		X	X	X							X							
	Vendor products									X	X					X			X			
	Public/private partnership																	X		X		
	Continuous quality improvement																	X	•			•
	Quality assurance																			•	•	

X = characteristic of program.
• = most emphasized feature of program.

1. Kowal (1997)
2. Wilson-Pessano et al. (1987); Wilson et al. (1993)
3. Forshee et al. (1998)
4. Wilson et al. (1996)
5. Griffin et al. (1989); Shields et al. (1990)
6. Moe et al. (1992)
7. McNabb et al. (1985)
8. Lewis et al. (1984)
9. Buchner et al. (1998)
10. Plaut et al. (1996)
11. Zieger et al. (1991)
12. Greineder et al. (1995)
13. Greineder et al. (1999)
14. Kropfelder (1996)
15. Stevens & Weiss-Harrison (1993)
16. Trubitt (1999)
17. Goonan et al. (1993)
18. Terry (1997)
19. Ellenbecker et al. (1998)
20. Wilson et al. (1998)
21. Ludwig-Beymer & Greene (1999)

dysfunction in all functional classes, including asymptomatic patients (Agency for Health Care Policy and Research [AHCPR], 1994; Cohn et al., 1986, 1991; CONSENSUS Trial Study Group, 1987; Pfeffer et al., 1992; The SOLVD Investigators, 1991, 1992). ACE inhibitors, in fact, appear to be the only therapy demonstrated to slow left-ventricular dysfunction and improve survival in CHF patients (Cohn, 1996; Follath, Cleland, Klein, & Murphy, 1998; Parmley, 1998; Young, Gheorghiade, Uretsky, Patterson, & Adams, 1998). Hydralazine isosorbide dinitrate is recommended for patients with systolic dysfunction who are intolerant of ACE inhibitors (Agency for Health Care Policy and Research (AHCPR), 1994; Cohn et al., 1986, 1991; ICSI, 1998). Second only to ACE inhibitor therapy is the recognized importance of diuretic use in patients with both systolic and diastolic dysfunction (AHCPR, 1994; Funke Kupper et al., 1986; Sigurd, Olesen, & Wennevold, 1975; Topol, Traill, & Fortuin, 1985; Whight, Morgan, Carney, & Wilson, 1974).

Other evidence-based pharmacological management guidelines include digoxin for patients with atrial fibrillation, third heart sound, or left ventricular dilation (AHCPR, 1994; Arnold et al., 1980; Lee et al., 1982; Packer et al., 1993) and beta-blockers for patients whose symptoms persist after the use of ACE inhibitors (Australia/New Zealand Heart Failure Research Collaborative Group, 1997; Packer et al., 1996; Waagstein et al., 1993).

The evidence for nonpharmacological therapies for CHF treatment is not as strong as that for pharmacotherapies, although recommendations exist. A sodium-restricted diet, sometimes with fluid restriction, is recommended for most patients (Dracup et al., 1994). It is also recommended that patients pursue a moderate exercise program after adequate screening (AHCPR, 1994; Belardinelli, Georgiou, Scocco, Barstow, & Purcaro, 1995; Coats et al., 1992; Dracup et al., 1994; Sullivan & Hawthorne, 1996), reduce stress (Beary, Benson, & Klemchuk, 1974; Mandle, Jacobs, Arcari, & Domar, 1996), and monitor daily weight gain (AHCPR, 1994; Dracup et al., 1994). Despite the existence of a well-established set of guidelines for CHF management, evidence suggests that compliance among practitioners with these guidelines is low (Rich, 1999; Wilkes et al., 1999). Patient compliance with recommended regimens is also frequently poor (AHCPR, 1994; Wilkes et al., 1999).

Because management of CHF involves a complex set of factors, including pharmacological, dietary, and behavior modification, and because CHF is rarely the sole health condition experienced by the patient, multidisciplinary team management of CHF patients has been proposed (Rich, 1999). Rich (1999) conducted a thorough review of the peer-reviewed articles on multidisciplinary management of CHF patients that were published between 1983 and 1998. In his review of 10 observational and six randomized controlled trials of multidisciplinary care, Rich (1999) comments on a "striking consistency in the reported findings" regarding the impact of multidisciplinary care: All of the studies demonstrated a decrease in hospital utilization among the treated populations. These studies also demonstrated varying levels of improved QoL, patient knowledge, functional status, patient compliance, and cost savings (Rich, 1999). Several of the studies included in the Rich (1999) review are also included in Appendix C. Of the studies contained in our reviews, those reported by Venner and Seelbinder (1996), Rich et al. (1993, 1995, 1996), Lasater (1996), Paul (1997), West et al. (1997), Urden (1998), Barrella and Monica (1998), Wilkes et al. (1999) and Pugh et al. (1999) describe multidisciplinary team management of CHF.

One of the problems that Rich (1999) highlights in his review of multidisciplinary interventions for CHF is the difficulty in pinpointing the specific aspects of these multifaceted interventions that actually affect patient outcomes. Rich (1999) also notes that the multidisciplinary interventions were implemented primarily in academic health centers, and the generalizability of these interventions to other settings is unknown.

Memberwide Interventions for CHF Management in MCOs

We did not find any studies describing chronic illness management interventions for CHF at the memberwide level that had a direct connection to MCOs. As described below, all interventions for CHF reported in MCOs occurred at the programwide level. Hospital-based interventions dominate the field of CHF disease management studies. Because they generally are not linked to the CHF population of a specific MCO, these hospital-based programs are classified below as interventions that serve an unknown population denominator.

CHF Management Interventions in MCOs at the Programwide Level

Wilkes et al. (1999) evaluated a comprehensive CHF management program at Kaiser Permanente of South San Francisco that had three components: (a) a CHF clinical pathway, (b) a patient-education module, and (c) a case management system. Only high-risk CHF patients (those with an ER visit or a hospital admission) were enrolled in the program. Management of patients in the Kaiser program began during the inpatient episode, where patients received consults from nutritional, pharmacy, social, and physical therapy services. Patients seen in the ER without a hospital admission were referred directly to a case manager. Patients received at least one home-care visit and were followed by a case manager who arranged outpatient visits, provided follow-up care, and scheduled patients for a series of five 2-hour educational classes (Wilkes et al., 1999). Instructional materials developed for the program were translated into several languages (both written and oral) to accommodate the culturally diverse patient population. Patient phone calls by the case manager were made once every 10 days until the patient was stabilized and once monthly thereafter. Case managers maintained frequent contact with patients' physicians, and provider education was used to increase adherence of prescribing practices to established guidelines (Wilkes et al., 1999).

The Kaiser program was evaluated with the first 252 enrolled patients. Hospital admissions among case-managed patients decreased 22.7% in the first 18 months of the program. CHF admission rates for program enrollees decreased from 1.44 per 100 case-managed members to 1.11 per 100 case-managed members in the 2 ½ years following program initiation. Total hospital admission rates for all other diagnoses did not change during the same time period. During this time period, average length of stay in the enrolled population decreased from 3.9 to 3.4 days, a decrease of 12.8%. The 5-day readmission rate for program enrollees decreased from 7.5 per 100 discharged to 4.0 per 100 discharged, a 46.7% decrease, 2 ½ years after program initiation. ER visits for the enrolled population decreased 21.7% over this time period, with a concomitant increase in outpatient visits of 3.2%. This increase in outpatient visits represented visits to the nurse case manager, however, not to cardiologists or primary-care physicians (Wilkes et al., 1999).

Wilkes et al. (1999) reported that ACE-inhibitor use increased from a baseline of 62.6% to 70.3% 2 years after implementation. Three years after implementation, this rate was 93%. Survey results indicated a high degree of patient satisfaction with educational classes; patients developed a better understanding of their disease and medications (Wilkes et al., 1999). In a survey of physician satisfaction with the program, to which two thirds of physicians responded, more than 80% reported that the program assisted them in managing care for their patients. About 77% of responding physicians reported that they received timely correspondence from their patients' case managers.

West et al. (1997) reported the results of a CHF management intervention at the programwide level that was conducted exclusively with managed care enrollees. The MULTIFIT intervention, a nurse-managed, physician-supervised, home-based management program for recently hospitalized CHF patients was implemented at Kaiser Permanente Medical Center in Hayward, California. Nurse case managers educated patients on various aspects of illness management according to clinical practice guidelines. Telephone contact with patients was maintained weekly by the nurse case manager for 6 weeks. This period of intensive communication was repeated if the patient experienced an ER visit or hospitalization. Patients whose condition remained stable after 6 weeks received phone contact every 2 to 4 weeks for an additional 18 weeks (West et al., 1997).

West et al. (1997) reported significant decreases in general medical visits, cardiology visits, and ER visits in the 6 months following implementation of the intervention compared to the 6 months prior. Hospitalization rates for CHF declined 87% in the 6 months following the intervention, and total hospitalization rates declined 74%. Patients reported significant increases in physical activity in the 6 months following implementation of the intervention (West et al., 1997).

The West et al. (1997) study suffers from two limitations that make generalizability of results extremely difficult. First, only 51 patients were included in the evaluation. Second, these patients were selected from a much larger potentially eligible population. During the time period selected for screening potential program participants, 291 patients were hospitalized for CHF. Of these patients, 238 (or 82%) were excluded from the study primarily because of comorbidities (e.g., patients with acute myocardial infarction within 8 weeks, valvular or myocardial obstructive disease, uncontrolled angina, or "other significant" comorbid conditions were excluded from analysis). Thus, the 51 patients who eventually participated in the intervention may have been those more likely to agree to participate or may have been preferentially selected for participation for other reasons.

Interventions for CHF Management With Unknown Population Denominators

The majority of CHF interventions take place in hospital settings, beginning while the patient is an inpatient and continuing after discharge. In fact, of the 15 interventions included in Appendix C, 12 take place in hospital settings and all but 1 of these hospital-based interventions (Topp, Tucker, & Weber, 1998) focus, for the most part, on an outpatient component that begins following hospital discharge. It is difficult, in these cases, clearly to identify the connection between these interventions and managed care populations.

There are two primary reasons why the bulk of CHF interventions are initiated in hospital settings. First, focusing an intervention on the highest risk patients (those who have been hospitalized or have used the ER) may provide the best opportunity to effect change in subsequent health outcomes and service utilization. Given finite resources and a high disease prevalence, it may make practical sense to focus interventions on those patients with the most severe CHF or those patients whose symptoms have led them to seek acute care.

A second explanation is based on the financial incentives faced by hospitals. Because most CHF patients are Medicare beneficiaries, hospitals may initiate CHF management programs in an effort to release patients quickly and/or to prevent costly readmission of patients. Payment for CHF hospitalizations is Diagnosis Related Groups-based for Medicare patients and, if a patient is readmitted for the same condition within 30 days, the hospitalization is considered part of the original episode. Hospitals, then, may initiate CHF management programs in an effort to reduce the overall costs of CHF hospitalizations to their institutions by preventing readmission.

Many hospital-based outpatient CHF management interventions, however, continue patient care well beyond 30 days after discharge, indicating that other factors drive the adoption of CHF management programs by hospitals. Of the hospital-based studies identified in this review, Lasater (1996), Venner and Seelbinder (1996), Paul (1997), Barrella and Monica (1998), Urden (1998), and Pugh et al. (1999) report on programs where outpatient management of discharged CHF patients continued beyond 30 days.

Hospital-based interventions for CHF are included in our review because they are the predominant form of disease management for CHF and because MCO patients are treated in the same hospitals as fee-for-service patients in most markets. Chronic illness management programs for CHF coordinated by hospitals may not be centrally organized or motivated by a single MCO, but patients enrolled in MCOs are presumably included in CHF management programs. A particular hospital may be part of an integrated care-delivery system or it may be that the existence of a CHF management program in a hospital setting influences an MCO to contract with a particular hospital. Actions taken by a hospital to improve its performance in the area of CHF may make it a more attractive source of care to both patients and contracting MCOs.

Not included in our review are studies of interventions for chronic illness conducted in Veterans' Administration settings because these settings do not serve managed care enrollees. More so than in diabetes, asthma, or arthritis, however, VA medical centers have been the setting for studies of CHF management interventions. Studies of CHF interventions in VA settings have included an increased role for nurse practitioners in care (Cintron, Bigas, Linares, Aranda, & Hernandez, 1983), the use of case managers (Fitzgerald, Smith, Martin, Freedman, & Katz, 1994), implementation of a home-monitoring system (Shah, Der, Ruggerio, Heidenreich, & Massie, 1998), and increased access to primary care for patients (Weinberger, Oddone, & Henderson, 1996). In addition, the establishment of a cardiomyopathy clinic in a VA medical center has been reported in the literature (Smith, Fabbri, Pai, Ferry, & Heywood, 1997).

Summary

No memberwide interventions for CHF management in clearly defined managed care settings were identified in the peer-reviewed literature. As described above, the literature in CHF management is dominated by hospital-based interventions, for which a clear connection to

MCOs is difficult to determine, as is the eligible patient population. Because the majority of interventions are hospital-based (and focus on currently or recently hospitalized patients), most CHF disease management efforts are geared toward the most severely ill patients.

Of the CHF programs reviewed, those interventions that demonstrated effective disease management in the populations enrolled in the intervention shared two common features. First, successful interventions employed nurse case managers as a part of a multidisciplinary team for patient care. Second, successful interventions provided patients with easy avenues for communication with providers (nurses, case managers, physician) in the case of worsening symptoms. It appears that the availability of care providers by phone allows patients to avoid unnecessary visits to the ER.

A recurring weakness in the literature regarding CHF management programs is the failure of studies to provide comprehensive evaluations of outcomes. A large number of the hospital-based programs noted here focus primarily on descriptions of the CHF management intervention. Other study limitations are listed in Appendix C. Literature reviewed regarding CHF management programs is presented in Appendix C. Table 6.4 describes the specific features of these interventions.

Cardiovascular Disease

The management of hypertension, dyslipidemia, and anticoagulation are similar in that each involves a specific outcome target (blood-pressure level, cholesterol level, or prothrombin time), and medication titration typically is used to achieve therapeutic outcome goals. The management guidelines for the treatment of hypertension and dyslipidemia that are most frequently employed are those of the Joint National Committee on Detection, Evaluation, and Treatment of High Blood Pressure and the National Cholesterol Education Project. These guidelines provide recommendations for lifestyle and medication management of elevated cholesterol and blood pressure. Management of anticoagulation follows titration recommendations based on measured bleeding times and is highly dependent on close patient monitoring.

(text continues on p. 150)

Table 6.4 Components of Congestive Heart Failure Management Programs

| | | Reference |
| | | Outpatient Program | | | | | | Hospital Program | | | | | | | |
Level of Focus	Characteristic	1	2	3	4	5	6	7	8	9	10	11	12	13	14
Patient	Patient education	X		X	•	X	X	X	X	X	X	X	X	X	
	Automated patient reminders														
	Computer interface for patients—high level											X			
	Patient-specific written management plan												X		
Provider	Provider education												X		X
	Physician profiling							X							
	Automated physician reminders														
	Guidelines/protocols	X	X	X			X	X		X	X	X	X	X	X
	Computer interface for provider—high level	X	X												
System	Multidisciplinary team		X	X		•	•	X	X	X	X	X	X		
	Nurse case management	X	•	•			X	•	•	•	X	X	X		
	Mini-clinic or dedicated day							X							
	Nurse-managed mini-clinic	•									•	•			
	Pharmacist as care provider											X			
	Alternative approaches to on-site contact	X	X	X		X	X	X	X			X	X	X	
	Nurse home visits	X		X		X	X						•		

		Reference												
		Outpatient Program				Hospital Program								
Level of Focus	Characteristic	1	2	3	4	5	6	7	8	9	10	11	12	13	14
	Formal relationships with external resources														
	Referral to specialist														
	Carve-outs	X													
	Special management of complex cases	X	X			X							X		
	Vendor products														
	Public/private partnership														
	Continuous quality improvement														•
	Quality assurance														

X = characteristic of program.
• = most emphasized feature of program.

Outpatient Programs
1. Brass-Myndarse (1996)
2. West et al. (1997)
3. Wilkes et al. (1999)

Hospital-Based Programs
4. Clark et al. (1992)
5. Rich et al. (1993, 1995, 1996)
6. Venner & Seelbinder (1996)
7. Urden (1998)
8. Pugh et al. (1999)
9. Topp et al. (1998)
10. Lasater (1996)
11. Paul (1997)
12. Barella (1998)
13. Gattis et al. (1999)
14. Rosenstein (1997)

Gerber (1997) argues that three motivating forces have led to increased chronic illness management efforts for dyslipidemia in managed care settings. First, market consolidation of delivery systems makes population-wide chronic illness management feasible. Second, published lipid management guidelines provide clear goals for therapy. Third, employer demand for high-quality care from MCOs has led to increased chronic illness management efforts in this area (Gerber, 1997).

Jacobs (1998) makes a similar argument regarding the management of hypertension by MCOs. According to Jacobs (1998), hypertension control is an area ripe for interventions by MCOs for several reasons: Hypertension is a common condition with defined risk strata; evidence-based, externally published guidelines exist for the management of hypertension; and the complications of the condition are preventable with proper management. Finally, lifestyle modification is a major method of disease management, making hypertension a prime target for population-wide disease management efforts (Jacobs, 1998).

More so than lipid or hypertension management, the intensive management of anticoagulation in patients is imperative for care systems. The Agency for Healthcare Research and Quality has reported that underuse of anticoagulant therapy among atrial fibrillation patients leads to 40,000 preventable strokes annually (Chiquette, Amato, & Bussey, 1998). Excessive anticoagulation of patients can lead to fatal bleeding events. The severe impact of mismanagement in population anticoagulation has led the American College of Chest Physicians to conclude that failure to use anticoagulation clinics in patient management increases provider legal liability (Chiquette et al., 1998; McIntyre, 1995). The establishment of anticoagulation management clinics, in fact, is not a new phenomenon ushered in by the proliferation of managed care. Anticoagulation management clinics have been in existence since the late 1970s, generally predating the development of hypertension and lipid management clinics.

For all three conditions, ample clinical evidence demonstrates that proper medical management can reduce disease mortality, morbidity, and costs (Chiquette et al., 1998; Garabedian-Ruffalo, Gray, Sax, & Ruffalo, 1985; Gerber, 1997; O'Connor et al., 1999). For hypertension and dyslipidemia, however, evidence suggests that adherence to disease management guidelines is universally poor (Cofer, 1997; Gerber, 1997; O'Connor et al., 1999).

Given the similarities among management needs for hypertension, dyslipidemia, and anticoagulation therapy, it is not surprising that chronic illness management strategies for these conditions generally share a common design: Care is managed by a nurse or pharmacist who oversees patient education and medication titration, while remaining in contact with the patient's primary-care physician.

Memberwide Interventions for Cardiovascular Disease Management in MCOs

Of the studies reviewed for hypertension, dyslipidemia, and anticoagulation management, two hypertension studies were conducted at the memberwide level. Pheley et al. (1995) described a long-standing nurse-managed hypertension screening and management program at Park Nicollet Medical Center in Minneapolis, Minnesota, which served primarily HMO patients under risk-based contracts. All patients who received care at the medical center had access to the program, which was originally established in 1972. The management program included hypertension screening, patient education, close monitoring of blood pressure by a nurse manager, and an automated system of patient appointment and medication reminders.

In a study of 200 patients enrolled in the program, Pheley et al. (1995) reported a significant improvement in the number of patients with blood pressure in control 12 months after enrollment. However, the program experienced an extremely high dropout rate; nearly 49% of patients left the program before the 12-month assessment date. In addition, generalizability is further limited because the medical center serves a predominantly white, middle-class, suburban population.

O'Connor et al. (1999) described the implementation of a hypertension management program in four HealthPartners (Minnesota) clinics. One site was a family practice clinic in a medium-size town with four family-practice physicians. The other three clinics were part of an eight-clinic system in St. Paul, Minnesota, and each had three family-practice physicians. The intervention was at the system level and included the implementation of hypertension management guidelines through the education of providers, the development of blood-pressure measurement and patient phone-call flow sheets, and use of a computerized patient-reminder system. The intervention also included the use of a CQI team to oversee implementation of the program in each clinic and improvements in documentation of patient care.

O'Connor et al. (1999) reported statistically significant improvements both in the proportion of patients achieving target blood-pressure levels and in average systolic and diastolic blood-pressure levels. In multivariate analysis controlling for age, gender, and number of outpatient visits, the implementation of the program was a significant predictor of the number of patients with blood pressure in control (O'Connor et al., 1999). The authors reported that the intervention led to an increased number of outpatient visits by patients, both to physicians and to nurse practitioners. An increase in costs associated with additional outpatient visits was anticipated and was expected to be short-term in nature (O'Connor et al., 1999).

The O'Connor et al. (1999) study may suffer from selection bias at the clinic level. The included clinics were those that had expressed particular interest in guidelines implementation and were the practice sites of physicians who were involved in large-scale guidelines development initiatives for the Institute for Clinical Systems Integration (ICSI), a Minnesota consortium of health care leaders with a major guidelines-implementation initiative under way. Success in these clinics, therefore, may not be generalizable to other, less motivated sites.

Cardiovascular Management Interventions in MCOs at the Programwide Level

Studies of interventions for CVD have been undertaken at the programwide level by MCOs (where not all members of the eligible patient population were enrolled in the intervention). Interventions for the management of hypertension, dyslipidemia, anticoagulation, and other cardiovascular conditions are dominated by the nurse- or pharmacist-managed outpatient clinic model. These clinics are primarily focused on medication titration and behavior modification. The predominant form of outcome evaluation for these programs has been the assessment of clinical outcome indicators.

For hypertension management interventions, the clinical outcomes of interest are the proportion of treated patients whose blood pressure is in control and the average change in blood-pressure levels among patients. For interventions focused on management of anticoagulation, the avoidance of adverse events (major and minor hemorrhagic events) and clinically evaluated bleeding rates (prothrombin times or INRs) are the relevant clinical outcome measures.

The success of hyperlipidemia management interventions is gauged primarily by decreases in cholesterol levels among treated patients. DeBusk et al. (1994) reported significantly lower cholesterol levels among intervention-group patients as compared to controls in a trial of a case-management intervention for recently hospitalized acute myocardial infarction (AMI) patients undertaken by five Kaiser Permanente medical centers in the San Francisco Bay area. Other direct measures of patient outcomes, such as the occurrence of ER visits or hospitalizations, have been used less frequently as indicators of program success, likely because the failure to control blood pressure or lipid levels seldom leads to immediate hospitalization or ER visits.

Measures of the process of care delivery to patients with hypertension and other CVDs have been used to evaluate chronic illness management interventions for these conditions. DeBusk et al. (1994) reported a significant increase in the proportion of patients receiving guidelines-recommended lipid-lowering medications among intervention-group patients following implementation of a case-management program of recently hospitalized AMI patients enrolled in five San Francisco Kaiser Permanente clinics.

Improvements in patient behaviors also are considered important outcomes in the management of hypertension and hyperlipidemia. DeBusk et al. (1994) reported significant increases in smoking cessation among patients enrolled in a case-management program for recently hospitalized AMI patients as compared to usual care controls.

Cardiovascular Disease Management With Unknown Population Denominators

As in the case of CHF, a great number of the chronic illness management interventions for hypertension and other CVDs occur in hospital settings. Interventions for hypertension and other cardiovascular conditions that took place in hospital settings are included in our literature review (Appendix D) because they potentially encompassed managed care enrollees. Hospital-based interventions for hypertension are described by Cantor, Morisky, Green, Levine, and Salkever (1985), Jones,

Jones, and Katz (1987b), Clark et al. (1992), and Schultz and Sheps (1994). Hospital-based anticoagulant management intervention studies are reported by Bussey, Rospond, Quandt, and Clark (1989), Seabrook, Karp, Schmitt, Bandyk, and Towne (1990), Becker et al. (1994), and Conte, Kehoe, Nielson, and Lodhia (1986). Chima, Miller-Kovach, Zeller, Cook, and Schupp (1990) and La Forge and Thomas (1996) presented hospital-based interventions for lipid management, and Anderson, Nangle, and Alexander (1997) described a systemwide intervention that focused on the management of all types of CVD at the hospital level.

Of the hospital-based interventions, only Seabrook et al. (1990) described an intervention that enrolled all eligible patients in the hospital setting into the chronic illness management program: a hospital-based anticoagulation program in which all patients hospitalized in an academic hospital (not identified by the authors) who required long-term anticoagulant therapy were referred to a nurse-managed anticoagulation clinic. Patients received educational information from a nurse prior to discharge from the hospital. Patient prothrombin bleeding times were recorded one to three times per week until the therapeutic warfarin dosage was attained. Nurse follow-up continued through phone contact and continued bleeding-time measurements. Noncompliant patients were referred to their primary-care physician for follow-up. No anticoagulant-related deaths or venous thrombotic events occurred in the study population during follow-up. The complication rate in the population was 3.2 events per 1,000 patient-months for minor hemorrhagic complications and 5.3 events per 1,000 patient-months for major bleeding events. No statistical analysis was conducted by Seabrook et al. (1990), and no comparison time period or population was presented, making it difficult to gauge the relative success of this program. The program is the only anticoagulation management study occurring at the memberwide level that was reported in the literature. The program was a hospital-based intervention, however, making the total eligible patient population difficult to identify from the perspective of evaluating management for managed care patients.

As in the case of CHF, several studies of hypertension and other cardiovascular interventions have taken place in VA settings: Aucott et al. (1996) described a guidelines-based hypertension management program introduced in two Cleveland VA clinics; Garabedian-Ruffalo et al.

(1985) described a pharmacist-managed anticoagulation clinic that was instituted in a Long Beach, California, VA medical center; and Brosnan (1996) described a similar clinic at a West Los Angeles VA medical center. Studies regarding interventions undertaken at VA medical centers are not included in this review.

Summary

In the literature we reviewed, successful hypertension and lipid management clinics share two common features. First, they use established external guidelines for care management, particularly medication management. Second, they tend to use nurses or pharmacists to oversee patient care, frequently in the context of a "dedicated day" or miniclinic.

The few evaluations of interventions for cardiovascular illness management share common methodological and design flaws. For example, their results are based on extremely small sample sizes or on large samples that have been cut into several small treatment arms. In addition, selection bias in the form of volunteer and exclusion bias limits generalizability. Finally, it is difficult to determine how patients were assigned to treatment or control groups in many cases. If patients who were referred to, or chose to attend, intervention programs are more or less likely to achieve favorable outcomes than those assigned to control-group status, it is problematic to generalize the results of the intervention to a memberwide population. Additional study limitations are noted in Appendix D.

Literature reviewed that relates to hypertension and other CVD management interventions is presented in Appendix D. Details of specific intervention characteristics are provided in Tables 6.5, 6.6, and 6.7.

Arthritis

An estimated 14.5% of the U.S. population is affected by osteoarthritis, rheumatoid arthritis, systemic lupus erythematosus, ankylosing spondylitis, or some other type of arthritis or connective tissue disorder (Hirano, Laurent, & Lorig, 1994). Osteoarthritis is the most

(text continues on p. 162)

Table 6.5 Components of Hypertension Management Programs

Level of Focus	Characteristic	\multicolumn{8}{c}{Reference}
		1	2	3	4	5	6	7	8
Patient	Patient education	•	•	•	X	X	X	X	X
	Automated patient reminders				X		X		
	Computer interface for patients—high level								
	Patient-specific written management plan								
Provider	Provider education				X	X			
	Physician profiling								
	Automated physician reminders				•				
	Guidelines/protocols							X	
	Computer interface for provider—high level							X	
System	Multidisciplinary team		X			•			
	Nurse case management					X			
	Mini-clinic or dedicated day								
	Nurse-managed mini-clinic						•	•	
	Pharmacist as care provider								
	Alternative approaches to on-site contact								X
	Nurse home visits								
	Formal relationships with external resources								X
	Referral to specialist								

156

Level of Focus	Characteristic	Reference							
		1	2	3	4	5	6	7	8
	Carve-outs								
	Special management of complex cases								
	Vendor products								
	Public/private partnership								•
	Continuous quality improvement				X	X			
	Quality assurance								

X = characteristic of program.
• = most emphasized feature of program.

1. Cantor et al. (1985)
2. Jones et al. (1987b)
3. Clark et al. (1992)
4. O'Connor et al. (1999)
5. Christianson et al. (1997)
6. Pheley et al. (1995)
7. Schultz & Sheps (1994)
8. Gerber & Stewart (1998)

Table 6.6 Components of Anticoagulation Management Programs

| Level of Focus | Characteristic | \multicolumn{5}{c}{Reference} |
		1	2	3	4	5
Patient	Patient education		X	X	X	X
	Automated patient reminders					
	Computer interface for patients—high level					
	Patient-specific written management plan		X			
Provider	Provider education					
	Physician profiling					
	Automated physician reminders					
	Guidelines/protocols		X			
	Computer interface for provider—high level		X			
System	Multidisciplinary team					
	Nurse case management					
	Mini-clinic or dedicated day	•		X	X	X
	Nurse-managed mini-clinic		•			
	Pharmacist as care provider			•	•	•
	Automated physician and patient reminders					
	Alternative approaches to on-site contact	X	X		X	
	Nurse home visits					
	Formal relationships with external resources					

158

Level of Focus	Characteristic	Reference				
		1	2	3	4	5
	Referral to specialist					
	Carve-outs					
	Special management of complex cases					
	Vendor products					
	Public/private partnership					
	Continuous quality improvement					
	Quality assurance					

X = characteristic of program.
• = most emphasized feature of program.

1. Seabrook et al. (1990)
2. Becker et al. (1994)
3. Bussey et al. (1989)
4. Wilt et al. (1995)
5. Conte et al. (1986)

Table 6.7 Components of Other Cardiovascular Disease (CVD) Management Programs

		Reference					
		Other CVD				Lipids	
Level of Focus	Characteristic	1	2			1	2
Patient	Patient education	X	X	X			
	Automated patient reminders						
	Computer interface for patients—high level						
	Patient-specific written management plan						
Provider	Provider education		X				
	Physician profiling						
	Automated physician reminders						
	Guidelines/protocols		X	X			
	Computer interface for provider—high level		X				
System	Multidisciplinary team			•			
	Nurse case management	•					
	Mini-clinic or dedicated day		•				
	Nurse-managed mini-clinic			X			
	Pharmacist as care provider						
	Alternative approaches to on-site contact	X					
	Nurse home visits						

Level of Focus	Characteristic	Reference				
		Other CVD		Lipids		
		1	2		1	2
	Formal relationships with external resources		X			
	Referral to specialist					
	Carve-outs					
	Special management of complex cases					
	Patient-specific written management plan					
	Vendor products					
	Public/private partnership					
	Continuous quality improvement		•			

Quality assurance

X = characteristic of program.

• = most emphasized feature of program.

Other CVD:

1. DeBusk et al. (1994)
2. Anderson et al. (1997)

Lipids:

1. Chima et al. (1990)
2. La Forge & Thomas (1996)

prevalent form of arthritis, affecting nearly 16 million Americans. Rheumatoid arthritis is the second-most prevalent of the rheumatologic conditions (Bilodeau, 1995; Hirano et al., 1994). Among those older than 65, 49% of Americans are estimated to have arthritis, according to the National Health Interview Survey (Bilodeau, 1995). Our discussion here is limited to the management of osteo- and rheumatoid arthritis because they are the most prevalent forms of arthritis.

Coordinated illness management for patient populations with arthritis is not well-addressed in the peer-reviewed literature, either in the context of MCOs or non-managed care systems. Only patient education as a disease management strategy for arthritis has been investigated extensively, but evidence regarding the impact of patient education on health status emerging from this body of literature is mixed.

Extensive reviews of the literature regarding arthritis-education interventions and the management of arthritis have been conducted by Mullen, Laville, Biddle, and Lorig (1987), Hirano et al. (1994), Hawley (1995), and Goeppinger and Lorig (1997). In a meta-analysis of 15 clinical trials of psychoeducational arthritis interventions, Mullen et al. (1987) calculated a 16% decrease in perceived pain, a 22% decrease in depression, and an 8% improvement in disability status among pooled populations of intervention-group patients versus controls. Hirano et al. (1994) present an extensive review of the results of published and unpublished studies of arthritis-education interventions conducted between 1987 and 1991. They report that these interventions were universally successful in improving patient knowledge about arthritis, and most were successful at improving health behaviors among patients (Hirano et al., 1994). Mixed results are reported by Hirano et al. (1994) in their review of the impact of interventions on psychosocial outcomes, and little evidence of an improvement in objective measures of health status (sedimentation rate, painful joint counts, grip strength, stiffness, and mobility) appears in the literature (Hirano et al., 1994). Of the variety of indicators of health status used to measure program impact, perceived pain appears to be the only outcome indicator affected by educational interventions in the Hirano et al. (1994) review.

Hawley (1995) presents a similar set of mixed results regarding the impact of educational interventions on arthritis outcomes in a review of 34 clinical trials published between 1985 and 1995. Most interventions were able to increase patient knowledge about arthritis, and several studies demonstrated slight improvements in functional ability, self-efficacy, and depression among patients. Hawley (1995) notes, however, that functional status appeared to be more highly correlated with psychological status than with any educational intervention. Although most of the interventions demonstrated decreased pain in patients, perceptions of pain also may be related to other psychological and social factors. Hawley (1995) noted that Lorig et al. (1986) found that pain among control-group patients actually improved more than among intervention-group patients. Finally, Hawley (1995) found no evidence of improvements in objective health-status measures, including joint counts, sedimentation rates, or grip strength, as a result of educational interventions.

Patient-education interventions appear to increase patients' knowledge and self-efficacy, improve health behaviors, and decrease perceived pain. However, the connection between patient education for arthritis management and actual improvements in health status or management of arthritis remains largely undemonstrated. Because arthritis is a progressive condition, it could be argued that educational interventions for the disease cannot be expected to improve objective measures of health status (Hawley, 1995). Rather, improvements in patient self-efficacy, behavior, and perceived pain may be suitable end goals for arthritis management.

As demonstrated by the extensive reviews highlighted above, there are numerous studies examining various types of educational interventions for arthritis. The impact of group education on arthritis management has been investigated by Barlow and Barefoot (1996), Basler (1993), Berg, Alt, Himmel, and Judd (1985), Goeppinger, Arthur, Baglioni, Brunk, and Brunner (1989), and others. Cognitive-behavioral approaches to arthritis education also have been reported in the literature (Basler, 1993; Calfas, Kaplan, & Ingram, 1992; Keefe et al., 1996 O'Leary, Shoor, Lorig, and Holman 1988; Parker et al., 1988; Young, Bradley, & Turner, 1995).

Programs specifically designed for rheumatoid arthritis patients have been extensively examined by Lorish, Parker, and Brown (1985), Berg et al. (1985), Strauss et al. (1986), O'Leary et al. (1988), Parker et al. (1988), Lindroth, Bauman, Barnes, McCredie, and Brooks (1989), Neuberger, Smith, Black, and Hassanein (1993), Davis, Busch, Lowe, Taniguchi, and Djkowich (1994), Young et al. (1995), Lindroth, Bauman,

Brooks, and Priestley (1995), and Lindroth et al. (1997). Comparisons of arthritis programs taught by laypeople to those taught by professionals have been conducted by Cohen, Sauter, DeVellis, and DeVellis (1986), Lorig, Lubeck, Kraines, Seleznick, and Holman (1985), and Lorig et al. (1986). Wetstone, Sheehan, Votaw, Peterson, and Rothfield (1985) and Rippey et al. (1987) have investigated computer-based educational programs for arthritis patients. Arthritis-education programs designed specifically for low-income patients have been described by Bill-Harvey et al. (1989) and Mazzuca et al. (1997).

Because of its prominence in the field, the work of Lorig et al. in the area of arthritis self-management deserves special attention. Lorig and colleagues have investigated the connection between improvements in self-efficacy and changes in health status among arthritis patients. Lorig is also responsible for the creation of the Arthritic Self-Management Program, which has been implemented nationally by the Arthritis Foundation, as well as internationally (Hawley, 1995; Lorig, Gonzalez, Laurent, Morgan, & Laris, 1998 Lorig & Holman, 1989, 1993; Lorig, Mazonson, & Holman, 1993; Lorig et al., 1989). Several studies of the Arthritis Self-Management Program have been reported for multiple populations, but none of these have exclusively enrolled managed care populations. It is not clear to what extent these studies included patients enrolled in managed care arrangements. Current implementation of the program for multiple chronic illness populations in the Kaiser system, reported by Lorig et al. (1999), is the only reference in the literature to the use of the program in an MCO.

Arthritis Disease Management Interventions in MCOs at the Programwide Level

We identified only two studies in the literature that evaluated chronic illness management interventions for arthritis undertaken by MCOs. Both of these interventions were at the programwide level. Fries, Carey, and McShane (1997) reported the results of a by-mail arthritis self-management intervention that was implemented with three patient populations: patients enrolled in Group Health in Seattle, patients attending three Northern California rheumatology clinics, and patients involved in Healthtrac, a general health-education program, who self-identified as arthritic. The by-mail program included individually tailored, computer-generated letters and care recommendations, as well as an instructional handbook, relaxation tape, and exercise video. Individualized patient letters were generated at 3-month intervals for 6 months.

Intervention-group patients were compared to controls in each of the three patient populations. After 6 months, in all patient populations, intervention-group patients demonstrated significant improvements compared to baseline and compared to controls in function, global vitality, tender-joint count, exercise frequency, and self-efficacy. Both intervention-group patients and controls demonstrated significant improvements in pain (Fries et al., 1997). Six months after the intervention, intervention-group patients had significantly fewer doctor visits both compared to baseline and compared to controls. At 1 year, the intervention group members continued to improve in painful-joint count and exercise frequency (Fries et al., 1997). As with most educational interventions for arthritis, it is impossible to determine if the impact of the intervention lasted beyond 12 months. It is possible that interventions that rely on patient education alone may require refresher courses for patients at various intervals to maintain a positive impact on health status.

Schned et al. (1995) described a multidisciplinary team-care intervention for patients with early-stage rheumatoid arthritis that took place at Park Nicollet Clinic in Minneapolis, Minnesota, a clinic that serves primarily managed care enrollees. A multidisciplinary care team comprising a rheumatologist, mental health specialist, social worker, podiatrist, outpatient nurse, dietician, physical therapist, and occupational therapist met monthly to review all new patients enrolled in the program and quarterly to review all enrolled patients. Patients and family members participated in half-day education and management programs. Patients participated in a phone assessment to identify patient-specific problems. A detailed care plan was developed for each patient and updated continuously by providers (Schned et al., 1995).

Eligible patients were randomized into treatment and control groups. After 1 year, no differences were observed between treatment and control groups in painful-joint count, duration of morning stiffness, functional class, fatigue, physical activity, dexterity, pain, mobility, or the presence of nodules. Also, no difference between groups was observed in depression, life satisfaction, perception of helplessness, use of medications, number of outpatient visits, tests ordered, hospitalizations, and surgical procedures (Schned et al., 1995). In part, the intervention may have failed to produce detectable differences between treatment- and control-group patients because both groups were treated by the same physicians. Some spillover effect of the intervention may have influenced care for the control group. The Schned et al. (1995) study also suffered from the relative homogeneity of the population. The clinic served a predominantly white, middle class, relatively affluent population at the time of the intervention, limiting generalizability of results to more diverse populations.

Summary

Clearly, research regarding the effective management of arthritis in MCOs (as well as in non-managed settings) is limited. Multiple educational interventions for arthritis management have been reported in the literature but, in general, these interventions lack a clear connection to improved patient outcomes. The Fries et al. (1997) intervention described above appears to have improved patient health outcomes, but the sustainability of these improvements remains undetermined.

The difficulty in designing a disease management intervention for arthritis arises from a lack of clearly defined care guidelines or definitively identified methods of improving patient outcomes. Unlike CHF or diabetes, there has been little research that suggests that multidisciplinary care teams or dedicated clinic days, for example, improve patient outcomes. In the absence of a clear direction for illness management in arthritis, educating patients about their condition has received the greatest attention as a means for improving patient management.

The two studies reviewed for arthritis management are presented in Appendix E; the details of intervention characteristics are provided in Table 6.8.

Overall Summary and Conclusions

Usual care, delivered through MCOs or other kinds of health care arrangements, does not yield outcomes achieved by patients enrolled in

Table 6.8 Components of Arthritis Management Programs

Level of Focus	Characteristic	Reference 1	Reference 2
Patient	Patient education	•	X
	Automated patient reminders		
	Computer interface for patients—high level		
	Patient-specific written management plan		X
Provider	Provider education		
	Physician profiling		
	Automated physician reminders		
	Guidelines/protocols		
	Computer interface for provider—high level		
System	Multidisciplinary team		•
	Nurse case management		
	Mini-clinic or dedicated day		
	Nurse-managed mini-clinic		
	Pharmacist as care provider		
	Alternative approaches to on-site contact	X	X
	Nurse home visits		
	Formal relationships with external resources		
	Referral to specialist		X
	Carve-outs		
	Special management of complex cases		
	Vendor products		
	Public/private partnership		
	Continuous quality improvement		
	Quality assurance		

X = characteristic of program.
• = most emphasized feature of program.
1. Fries et al. (1997)
2. Schned et al. (1995)

efficacy studies. This provides an opportunity for disease management programs to improve patient outcomes. Efficacy studies identify interventions that can work, but the challenge is to develop techniques to deploy these interventions in managed care settings. These techniques are at the heart of the definition of managed care as a vehicle to influence the delivery of health services to a defined population.

As previously noted, it is no surprise that usual care does not deliver the same rate of improvement as efficacy studies. Efficacy studies involve volunteers, a group known to comply better and have better outcomes than nonvolunteers. Efficacy studies often are well funded and can support teams that actively encourage patients to comply with interventions. These teams follow protocols with regularly scheduled follow-up, in contrast to usual care, which frequently focuses on acute follow-up.

As detailed in Table 6.1 at the beginning of this chapter, we reviewed 89 studies but found only 5 that described an effective intervention that improved the health of a population with a specific chronic condition. Many studies were primarily descriptive, did not adequately define the population denominator, or had no comparative data analysis. Of the studies that defined the eligible population and identified an appropriate comparison group, most had the significant limitation of examining effects only on the patients within the program rather than on all eligible patients in a defined population. In other words, most studies looked at a programwide denominator rather than a memberwide denominator. It is possible that an intervention may show some benefit for the individuals within the program, but unless one understands the impact of the program on the denominator of patients who may potentially benefit, one cannot conclude that the program was effective in improving the health status of the broader group. Using only a programwide denominator raises the following issues:

- One cannot understand the impact on the potential pool of patients within a population who may benefit from the program. For referral programs, one often cannot discern the criteria used to refer patients to the program and what percentage of the eligible population was enrolled. A program enrolling 95% of the eligible population may be quite different than a program enrolling only 1% of an eligible population. Most studies of specialty clinics suffer from this problem.

- Studies of programwide interventions can exhibit selection or attrition bias. Patients who volunteer for the program may be different than patients who do not volunteer. Similarly, patients referred to programs may represent either more or less severely ill patients, depending on the program protocol. Also, patients who remain with the program throughout the study period may differ from early dropouts.
- A program that treats a small subset of patients within a defined population may not be economically sustainable when applied to the entire eligible population.

Because we found only a handful of effective interventions, we could not draw conclusions about which program components made a difference. In almost all cases, the research design of the published evaluations did not allow researchers to evaluate the effectiveness of individual components. Depending on the specific disease, most of the programs that we reviewed, and which seemed to have the most promise for future success, shared the following features:

Multidisciplinary team care with an increased role for nurses. In diabetes, see Joshi and Bernard (1999) and Legorreta et al. (1996). In CHF, see West et al. (1997) and Wilkes et al. (1999).

Implementation of care guidelines at the system level. In diabetes, see O'Connor et al. (1996), Ginsberg et al. (1998), Mazze et al. (1994), and Chicoye et al. (1998). In CHF, see West et al. (1997) and Wilkes et al. (1999). In CVD, see O'Connor et al. (1999) and Chima et al. (1990).

Patient education and involvement in the care process. In diabetes and asthma, see all interventions. In CHF, see Wilkes et al. (1999). In CVD, see Clark et al. (1992) and DeBusk et al. (1994). In arthritis, see Fries et al. (1997).

Nurse- or pharmacist-managed miniclinics. In asthma, see Greineder et al. (1995, 1999). In CVD, see Pheley et al. (1995), all anticoagulation interventions, and Chima et al. (1990).

A focus on high-risk populations. In diabetes, see Joshi and Bernard (1999) and Rubin et al. (1998). In asthma, see Wilson-Pessano et al. (1987), Wilson et al. (1993), Forshee et al. (1998), Wilson et al. (1996),

Griffin et al. (1989), Shields, Griffin, and McNabb (1990), McNabb et al. (1985), Lewis et al. (1984), Zeiger et al. (1991), and Greineder et al. (1995, 1999). In CHF, see West et al. (1997), Wilkes et al. (1999), and all hospital-based interventions. In CVD, see Jones et al. (1987b).

Solberg et al. (1997) wrote that "despite clear national guidelines, various examples of better care models, and multiple attempts to improve care, an effective process for facilitating and replicating diabetes care improvements in typical primary care practices has been elusive" (p. 582). The same could be said for the other chronic conditions included here. As Wagner (1997) emphasized, MCOs have the structural and systemic advantages that should enable them to manage chronic illness successfully, but there is little research evidence that these attributes have led to improved outcomes for patients on a wide scale.

Our review of the literature has demonstrated that at least some MCOs are attempting to manage care for chronically ill patients with diabetes, asthma, CHF, and cardiovascular conditions. A vast number of articles provide only descriptions of interventions. Although they are not included in our literature review, these publications are useful in understanding the different initiatives being undertaken by MCOs to treat patients with chronic illnesses. However, they do not establish, using accepted research standards, the impact of the programs on patient outcomes. Several of the studies that are included provide relatively informal evaluations of disease management programs based on preliminary findings and anecdotal evidence. Reports that "most physicians who directed patients to the program were pleased with results . . ." or general presentations of cost savings without explanation of how the sample was created, data gathered, and costs calculated permit only a limited assessment of how well a program worked.

It is also worth noting that most of the literature reviewed in this chapter fails to address the issue of sustainability of interventions. The evaluation of chronic illness intervention programs, when formally conducted, tends to occur over no more than 18 to 24 months following program implementation. Some of the hypertension studies reviewed are an exception to this. For the most part, however, the sustainability of promising interventions has not been demonstrated. In fact, in most cases, it was difficult to determine if an attempt was made to continue the intervention beyond the initial evaluation period. To achieve continuing success in disease management, interventions must be economically sustainable within the MCO. In addition, they must be sustainable from the perspective of physician and patient buy-in to the program.

Finally, patient satisfaction with, and acceptance of, disease management interventions has largely been ignored in the literature thus far. A few studies employ measurements of QoL as outcome indicators, but generally these measures are used when clinical improvements are either difficult to detect or are not realistically expected (as in the case of arthritis). This is despite research findings that suggest chronic illness management interventions require patient involvement and support if they are to achieve improvement in outcomes and be sustained. One of the primary criticisms of the DCCT is that, although it was successful in reducing the complications of diabetes in subjects, it required a level of patient diligence that may be unrealistic to expect outside of a clinical trial. Patient education and involvement in the care process have been recognized as key components of chronic illness management. Patient education has been included as part of many chronic illness management interventions, but this education comes in the form of what providers believe patients should know about their condition. Little work has investigated what patients want to know and to what degree they desire to be involved in their own care.

APPENDIX A: Literature Describing Diabetes Management Programs in Managed Care Organizations

Level of Focus	Reference	Setting/Population	Intervention	Results
Patient	Franz et al. (1995)	**Setting:** Three outpatient diabetes centers located in Minnesota, Florida, and Colorado **Population:** Programwide, with patients recruited through doctor referral, self-referral, or notices posted at clinics. Intervention group compared to randomized and nonrandom control groups ($N = 247$).	Medical Nutrition Therapy (MNT) is a guidelines-based nutrition therapy for diabetics consisting of three visits with a nutritionist over a 6-week period. The basic goals of MNT are to lower fat and energy intake, spread out food intake over the day, increase exercise, and improve food choice. The ultimate goal of the program is to improve glycemic control. Patients were randomized to the MNT program or to a single nutritionist visit at entry. Patients were also compared to a nonrandomized group of controls receiving no nutrition therapy.	1. Both the MNT group and patients receiving a single nutritionist visit experienced significant decreases in fasting blood glucose and HbA1c at each evaluation point (6 weeks, 3 months, and 6 months). 2. Total cholesterol in the MNT group decreased significantly at 3 and 6 months. Patients in the single nutritionist-visit group experienced a decrease in cholesterol at the 3 months evaluation point, but the levels rose again at 6 months. 3. Both the MNT and the single nutritionist-visit group experienced significant weight loss by 6 months, but no change in waist-to-hip ratio. 4. No change in glycemic control occurred in the nonrandomized control group receiving no nutrition counseling. No other outcome variables were measured for this group. **Limitations:** 1. Volunteer bias: Patients either self-referred in response to posted ads or were referred by a physician. 2. Short follow-up period (6 months) does not explore sustainability of intervention or its effects.

Level of Focus	Reference	Setting/Population	Intervention	Results

Patient	McNabb et al. (1993)	**Setting:** Endocrinology clinic of an inner-city medical center in Chicago, IL
		
		Population: Programwide, with nonrandomized usual-care control group from same setting, later entered into program ($N = 23$).
			PATHWAYS is a weight-loss program designed for inner-city black women with non-insulin dependent diabetes mellitus (NIDDM). The goal of PATHWAYS is to promote long-term weight loss and improve diabetic control. The 18-week program involved 12 weekly educational sessions followed by 6 weeks of reinforcement sessions. Instruction includes training in goal-setting, reading food labels, determining reasons for overeating, ordering in restaurants, and preparing food. Dietary recommendations are focused around American Diabetes Association (ADA) guidelines.	1. Intervention group patients lost a significant amount of weight (9 lbs by the 18-week follow-up point and an addition 0.8 lbs by the 1-year follow-up point, $p < .008$). The control group gained an average of 3 lbs by the 1-year follow-up point.
				2. The intervention group decreased mean HbA1c by 2.6% at the 18-week outcome point, but by 1 year, these levels had returned to their baseline value (12.8%). HbA1c levels for the control group were not provided.
				
				Limitations:
				  1. Extremely small sample size.
				  2. Consistent comparisons between controls and intervention group were not made (no HbA1c information available for controls).
				  3. The control group was not a randomized control group and may not be comparable to the intervention group.

Level of Focus	Reference	Setting/Population	Intervention	Results
Patient	Singer et al. (1995)	**Setting:** Harvard Community Health Plan, Boston, MA **Population:** Description of intervention only, no population used for evaluation.	Harvard Community Health Plan (HCHP) provides self-management education for diabetics from a multidisciplinary team. Most diabetics continue to receive care from their primary-care physician but receive education from a trained corps of certified diabetes educators and dieticians. A computerized system helps to coordinate education and care and generates reminders for patients about clinic and education appointments. One-on-one self-management education is combined with group education. HCHP has developed its own diabetes manual for patients and provides low-cost blood glucose-testing supplies for all patients to use at home. HCHP has partnered with LifeScan, which provides blood glucose-testing equipment to the plan and to patients at reduced cost. HCHP's ultimate goal is to provide home glucose-monitoring supplies to every diabetic patient at no cost.	1. No results presented. **Limitations:** 1. Description of intervention only; no evaluation presented. Not a scholarly/academic article.

Level of Focus	Reference	Setting/Population	Intervention	Results
Patient	McNabb et al. (1994)	**Setting:** Diabetes clinic of a large metropolitan children's hospital in Chicago, IL. **Population:** Programwide, with randomized usual-care controls taken from same setting ($N = 22$).	The In Control program is an educational intervention designed to improve self-management of insulin-dependent diabetes mellitus (IDDM) among children. The program consists of six weekly small-group sessions for children, with concurrent sessions for their parents. The goal of the program is to teach children to take control of their own diabetes management. Parents and children meet to discuss goal setting and to practice behavior change.	1. Children in the intervention group achieved significantly higher "responsibility scores" than children in the control group. Responsibility scores were determined through a parent questionnaire. 2. The frequency of performance of diabetes-care behaviors did not differ significantly between intervention and control-group children. 3. After controlling for baseline levels, HbA1c levels in the two groups did not differ significantly after the intervention. **Limitations:** 1. Results are dependent on parental report of child's behavior. 2. Small sample size. 3. Volunteer bias: of 76 eligible, only 24 participated.

Level of Focus	Reference	Setting/Population	Intervention	Results
Provider	Benjamin et al. (1999)	**Setting:** Baystate Medical Center, Tufts University School of Medicine, and its three urban primary-care sites in Springfield, MA **Population:** Programwide, with patients randomized to treatment or control group at the firm level. Each firm consists of a geographically separate group of practitioners, patients, and inpatient and outpatient facilities ($N = 144$).	The intervention consists of a problem-based educational tool for providers based on Staged Diabetes Management. Residents and physicians in the intervention firm researched various aspects of diabetes management independently and then came together for four 2-hour sessions to discuss improvement of diabetes care within the firm. Providers also met at 6 and 12 months for lunchtime sessions. Care protocols developed for the Staged Diabetes Management system were used as the core of clinical practice guidelines that were created by the group. The final products were a stepped-care guideline for glycemic control and other guidelines for improving adherence to standards of care for diabetic patients. Patients in both the intervention and control firms received care in the firm care system already in place at the Medical Center, which provided patients with multidisciplinary care.	1. At 9 months after the intervention, patients in the intervention group experienced a significant drop in HbA1c, whereas control groups demonstrated a slight increase. HbA1c levels did not change significantly between 9 and 15 months in either group. 2. Significantly more patients in the intervention group than in the control group demonstrated improvements in HbA1c over the time period. 3. Annual preventive screening rates for urine protein, retinopathy, and so on remained constant in the control clinic following implementation of the intervention but increased in the intervention firm. 4. Following the intervention, a greater number of patients in the intervention firm as compared to the control firm were moved to more aggressive forms of pharmacological therapy. Limitations: 1. Although the guidelines implementation at the firm level should affect all enrolled patients in diabetes, relatively small groups of patients from each firm were used for evaluation. 2. Providers in the intervention clinic did not use the clinical practice guidelines with patients if they felt that the guidelines were too strict for the particular patient and would lead to hypoglycemic episodes. 3. Differences between care environments in the two firms, or between the patient populations enrolled in the two firms, may have affected results.

Level of Focus	Reference	Setting/Population	Intervention	Results
Provider	Smith et al. (1998)	**Setting:** Mayo Clinic, Rochester, MN **Population:** Programwide, with comparison group from same setting ($N = 82$).	Diabetes Electronic Management System (DEMS) is an electronic medical record system used in real time by clinicians to aid in management of care for diabetic patients. Data regarding the patient's reason for clinic visits can be entered into the system just prior to the visit. Clinical information can be entered into the patient's record while the physician is meeting with the patient. DEMS records treatment goals and guidelines established by the patient and physician during the appointment. At the end of each visit, a paper record of all recorded information is printed and added to the patient's medical record file.	1. Patients whose physicians used the DEMS system had more foot examinations than those whose doctors used the paper record system. 2. DEMS patients had significantly higher criterion scores (a weighted sum of the frequency of various procedures) than paper record controls. 3. DEMS patients had a significantly higher number of blood-pressure measures and HbA1c tests than paper record controls. **Limitations:** 1. Only process measures are reported; there is no examination of impact on health outcomes. 2. No information is reported regarding cost to the system or physician response.
System	Abourizk et al. (1994)	**Setting:** St. Francis Hospital and Medical Center, Hartford, CT **Population:** Programwide, no comparison group ($N = 141$).	The intervention consisted of a reimbursable, outpatient referral Diabetes Care Clinic (DCC) that offers a 4-day treatment program for diabetics. The program emphasizes multidisciplinary care and instruction and maintains contact with the patient's primary-care physician.	1. Among the 69 patients, mean HbA1c fell from $9.97 \pm .28$ to $7.53 \pm .28$ after 12 months. HbA1c levels decreased in 84% of patients and remained the same in 16%. 2. HbA1c levels decreased more dramatically among those with higher initial levels. **Limitations:** 1. The treatment clinic is a referral center. It is not clear what the patient denominator is. 2. Of 137 patients treated in the clinic during the study period, only 69 were available for follow-up 8 months later and only 49 had complete follow-up data. The authors report no baseline differences between drop-outs and those who remained in the study population.

Level of Focus	Reference	Setting/Population	Intervention	Results
System	Sadur et al. (1999)	**Setting:** Kaiser Permanente Medical Care Program, Pleasanton, CA. **Population:** Programwide, with patients randomized to treatment or control group ($N = 185$).	The Diabetes Cooperative Care Clinic (DCCC) uses multidisciplinary team care led by a nurse educator. Patients in the intervention group entered the 6-month program and were then returned to care with their primary-care physician. Intervention consisted primarily of monthly 2-hour visits for 10 to 18 patients as a group. Patients were referred for additional education, screening, eye exams, and behavioral training as necessary. Nurse educators maintained telephone contact with patients between visits. Care team met regularly to discuss cases. At the end of the 6-month intervention, detailed notes and care plans were forwarded to patients' primary-care physicians.	1. After 6 months, there was a significant decrease in HbA1c levels among intervention-group patients as compared to controls. However, at 12 months, control-group patients' HbA1c levels decreased to intervention group levels. 2. Insulin and oral medication use increased in the intervention group but remained stable in the control group. 3. There was no difference between groups in satisfaction with care. 4. 18 months after the intervention, intervention-group hospital discharge rates were significantly lower than control-group rates. 5. During the 6 months of the intervention, outpatient visits to physicians among controls decreased by 17%; visits to nonphysicians increased eight-fold. **Limitations:** 1. The 12- and 18-month outcomes are contaminated because patients from the control group were entered into the intervention sometime near the 12-month time point. 2. No information on the cost of the intervention was provided.

Level of Focus	Reference	Setting/Population	Intervention	Results
System	Domurat (1999)	**Setting:** Kaiser Permanente, Harbor City, CA **Population:** Programwide, 2,617 nonrandomized intervention-group patients compared to 5,993 usual-care patients. Only "high-risk" patients are entered into the program.	The Diabetes Care System (DCS) includes care for high-risk diabetic patients by a multidisciplinary team with nurse case management. The intervention includes patient education, screening, and telemanagement. The DCS uses a systemwide diabetes registry to identify high-risk patients and track all visits, phone contact, and laboratory results. The computer system is also used for communication between providers. It is estimated that about 30% of patients (all high-risk) receive management through the DCS system.	1. Testing for HbA1c, lipids, and proteinuria occurred at significantly higher rates among intervention-group than usual-care patients. 2. Among those with more than one HbA1c in the intervention group: for those with HbA1c initially within target range, there was a significant increase in HbA1c; for those with initial levels above target, there was a significant decrease in HbA1c. Patients in usual care with initially elevated HbA1c levels also experienced a significant decrease in HbA1c over time. 3. There was no difference between intervention and usual-care groups in absolute level or change in HbA1c. 4. Blood pressure decreased significantly among those in the intervention group with initially high levels. No change in blood pressure occurred among usual-care patients. 5. Patients managed in the program long-term had significantly reduced hospitalization rates over time. **Limitations:** 1. The intervention and usual-care groups are not comparable, as the intervention group was comprised of high-risk, more severely ill patients. It is not clear, therefore, what comparisons presented by the authors represent. 2. The intervention group differed from the usual-care group in terms of age and gender (in addition to disease severity).

Level of Focus	Reference	Setting/Population	Intervention	Results
System	Aubert et al. (1998)	**Setting:** Two large clinics in the Jacksonville Health Care Group, the largest provider of health care services for the Prudential HealthCare HMO plan of Jacksonville, FL. **Population:** Programwide, with randomized control group from same setting ($N = 138$).	A nurse case manager follows a disease-management algorithm in this program. The program includes extensive patient education and quarterly follow-up appointments with a nurse case manager. Intervention-group patients initially met with a case manager and were taught blood glucose self-monitoring. At a 2-week follow-up visit, patient blood-glucose diaries were reviewed by the nurse and medications were adjusted. Patients were referred to a 5-week, 12-hour education class. The nurse case manager met regularly with the primary-care physician. Patients assigned to usual care were provided with blood glucose-testing supplies and encouraged to seek diabetes education.	1. After 12 months, the intervention group experienced a greater decrease in HbA1c level than the control group (–1.7% versus –0.6%, $p < .001$). 2. Fasting blood-glucose levels in the intervention group decreased by 48.32 mg/dL versus 14.6 mg/dL in the control group ($p < .003$). 3. There were no changes in either group in blood pressure, cholesterol, triglyceride levels, insulin dose, or weight. 4. Both groups reported increased perceived health status. 5. No significant differences between the groups emerged in emergency-room visits, outpatient visits, or low blood-sugar events. **Limitations:** 1. Exclusion bias and volunteer bias are potential issues: Only 208 of 545 identified diabetics were deemed eligible to participate in the study. Of these 208, 34% failed to appear for their first appointment. 2. Randomization was not successful. The intervention group had fewer minorities, more smokers, and more patients using insulin. 3. Initial average HbA1c levels were 8.8% in the intervention group and 8.4% in the usual-care group. This represents a relatively high level of good control and probably reflects the sampling process used.

Level of Focus	Reference	Setting/Population	Intervention	Results
System	Edelstein et al. (1993)	**Setting:** Beth Israel Hospital, New York City **Population:** Programwide, with control group from same setting identified retrospectively (N = 160 + control group of unknown size).	Nurse case management was used for hospitalized diabetic patients. The nurse case manager coordinates care from a multidisciplinary team and serves as a gatekeeper for care while the patient is in the hospital. The nurse case manager also provides diabetic education and is a contact for the patient after release.	1. The average length of stay in the intervention group was 4.14 days if diabetes was the primary diagnosis versus 9.9 days in the control group. The national average in 1990 was 7.8 days. 2. For patients with diabetes as the secondary diagnosis, the average length of stay was 10.7 days in the intervention group and 11.8 days in the control group. 3. At release, blood-glucose control was excellent in 28.7% of the intervention group, good in 26.9%, fair in 42.7%, and poor in 1.46%. No comparison to controls was provided for this outcome measure. **Limitations:** 1. Patients were only entered into the study if they did not have private physicians. 2. The control group was retrospectively matched to the intervention group, and matching by socioeconomic status was not done. 3. The size of the control group is unknown. 4. 1993 intervention-group data were compared to 1990 control-group data, which may be problematic when using length of stay as an outcome measure. 5. The analysis was not multivariate.

Level of Focus	Reference	Setting/Population	Intervention	Results
System	Graff et al. (1995)	**Setting:** Group Health Cooperative of Puget Sound, Seattle, WA **Population:** Memberwide, all diabetic patients who sought care at a particular Group Health of Puget Sound clinic ($N = 1,000$).	This was a pilot project to examine an expanded role for nurses in diabetes care. The goal of the program was to establish coordinated care for diabetics emphasizing a team approach. Nurses worked to improve accessibility to services and designed and evaluated programs for diabetics. Nurses were trained in case management and reported to physicians on the health of the treated population. A major part of the nurse's role involved education of clinic staff and physicians in diabetes-management techniques.	1. The nurse clinician reported to physicians that when diabetic patients were case-managed by a nurse, basic standards of diabetes care were met. 2. Nurse-clinician presentations resulted in increased interest among physicians in training their nurses to become case managers. 3. Nurse office visits increased in clinics where the nurse clinician had trained nurses in case management. **Limitations:** 1. No assessment of the impact of intervention on health outcomes is presented.
System	Peters et al. (1995)	**Setting:** Cedars-Sinai Medical Center in Southern California, an IPA contracting with 22 HMOs **Population:** Programwide, with patients referred to the service by primary-care provider. The study does not evaluate a single cohort of patients.	The Comprehensive Diabetes Care Service (CDCS) is a nurse-managed care program for diabetic patients; it includes patient reminders of appointments and laboratory tests combined with nurse management of care according to care protocols. Each nurse manager cares for a caseload of 250 diabetic patients and is supervised by a diabetologist. Diabetologists do not provide one-on-one care but rather manage the care team of nurse specialists. Thirty-two care protocols have been developed. Reporting of patient status to the primary-care doctor is included in management.	1. The authors conclude that over 4 years, 244 patients would have been hospitalized by other providers, had they not been enrolled in the intervention. This resulted in a hypothesized cost savings of $1.2 million over 4 years. Over this time period, program costs were $631,279. 2. In the first year of the program, HbA1c levels dropped from 12.5 ± 0.4 to 9.5 ± 0.2. **Limitations:** 1. This article was mainly a description of the program, not a formal evaluation. 2. It is not clear how the authors arrived at their estimates of the program's impact on avoided hospitalizations. 3. No statistical testing was included. 4. HbA1c's were only compared for the subset of patients who had the test from year to year.

Level of Focus	Reference	Setting/Population	Intervention	Results
System	Peters & Davidson (1998) Davidson (1997)	**Setting:** Cedars-Sinai Medical Center and a Los Angeles HMO **Population:** Programwide, with intervention patients referred by physicians compared with controls from a different setting ($N = 165$).	This intervention involves a nurse-managed Comprehensive Diabetes Care Services (CDCS) program at Cedars-Sinai Medical Center (see Peters et al., 1995, above). This description of the program places more emphasis on the contribution of computer-assisted management to the program. A computer database tracks patient appointments, automatically generates laboratory orders according to ADA guidelines, and generates reminder notices for patients until an event occurs. Patient appointments and laboratory testing are scheduled automatically according to ADA guidelines and patient medication status. The computer system is used to track laboratory results and store patient home blood glucose-monitoring results.	1. Intervention-group patients had significantly higher HbA1c levels at baseline, but by Year 1, their levels were significantly reduced, and they remained significantly lower through Year 3. 2. Total cholesterol did not change for control or intervention groups as a whole. Among those with high cholesterol only, there was a significant decrease in cholesterol levels among intervention-group patients but not among controls. 3. No differences between groups appeared in blood pressure, proteinuria, or microalbuminuria. 4. Process measures related to diabetic management were more favorable in the intervention group. 5. General QoL was similar in both groups. At baseline, the intervention group had worse diabetes-specific QoL than the control group. Diabetes-specific QoL improved in the intervention group but remained constant in the control group. **Limitations:** 1. The study was not multivariate. 2. The control group was from a different patient population than the intervention group. 3. 34% of intervention-group members were lost to follow-up because of a change in insurance provider.

Level of Focus	Reference	Setting/Population	Intervention	Results
System	Legorreta et al. (1996)	**Setting:** Two medical groups that contract to provide care to enrollees of Health Net, an HMO in Woodland Hills, CA. One site, a participating medical group (PMG), the other an IPA. **Population:** Programwide: The PMG site was compared to a control PMG site. Within the IPA, 13 physician office sites served as control sites. At each intervention site, 15 diabetic patients were selected randomly and entered into the program. All new diabetic patients at intervention sites were entered into the program ($N = 390$; 240 in the intervention group versus 150 controls).	Team care of diabetic patients was led by a nurse case manager or a physician assistant. This program was originally tested at Cedars-Sinai Medical Center. Nurses, physician assistants, and endocrinologists attended a 2-week training course at Cedars-Sinai Medical Center. Nurses and physician assistants used detailed care protocols. A computer information system was used to track patient appointments, send patient reminders, track laboratory testing, provide a database of patient records, and recommend medication dosing based on home blood-glucose monitoring. Providers at the intervention sites met quarterly with facilitators from Cedars-Sinai.	1. From baseline to the last HbA1c measurement (after a maximum of 28 months), patients in the intervention groups had significantly greater decreases in HbA1c levels than patients in the control groups. 2. The decrease in HbA1c levels was significantly greater among intervention-group patients at the PMG compared to intervention-group patients at the IPA. 3. At the intervention PMG site, 100% of patients were referred for a retinal exam, and 99.2% had documentation that the exam took place. At the intervention IPA sites, only 52% of patients had recorded referrals for eye exams, and only 11.4% had evidence that the exam occurred. **Limitations:** 1. The initial enrollment plan for the intervention sites did not result in enough participants, so after 6 months, physicians were allowed to enroll patients in the intervention nonrandomly. This resulted in selection bias. Patients with the worst-controlled diabetes were more likely to be enrolled in the program. 2. Fewer than 40% of patients at the two control sites had baseline HbA1c levels reported. 3. Comparable information regarding retinal examinations was not available for control-group members. 4. The authors note a high rate of staff turnover at one of the intervention sites. Replacement staff were trained in the protocol on site, rather than receiving training from Cedars-Sinai.

Level of Focus	Reference	Setting/Population	Intervention	Results
System	Geffner (1992)	**Setting:** Multiple settings **Population:** Programwide, with all patients enrolled in CIGNA's HMO and IPA-network plans eligible; referrals occurred at the primary-care physician's discretion.	Diabetes care clinics were available to diabetic patients enrolled in CIGNA Health Plan's staff-model HMOs. Clinics consisted of multidisciplinary care teams following care protocols. Referral to the clinics occurred at the primary-care provider's discretion. Patients had unlimited free access to educational programs, and each doctor visit was followed by a visit with a certified diabetic educator and a dietitian. CIGNA's IPA contracts with physicians who see HMO and fee-for-service patients in the diabetes clinics. Referral is under the control of primary-care physicians, who remain under financial risk with certain stop-loss provisions.	1. No results presented. **Limitations:** 1. Description of care program only. No formal evaluation was conducted.

Level of Focus	Reference	Setting/Population	Intervention	Results
System	Gerber et al. (1998)	**Setting:** Kaiser Permanente Southern California pharmacies **Population:** Programwide, randomization occurred at the pharmacy level. Patients could attend the pharmacy of their choice.	Pharmacists were used as care providers for high-risk patients. Pharmacists provided patient education to diabetics based on written protocols and contacted primary care providers if they anticipated self-management problems. Three models were compared: (a) the control model reflected pharmacy practice before implementation of state-mandated pharmacy consultations; (b) the state model followed new state-mandated requirements for written or verbal counseling by pharmacists for all new medications; (c) the Kaiser model expanded the state requirements by focusing service on high-risk patients, providing patient education and follow-up, contacting the primary-care physician if perceived problems arose, and reviewing medication compliance based on frequency of medication refills.	1. Among insulin-only users, filling prescriptions in the state-model system significantly reduced total medical cost (by 7.8% for each prescription filled) compared to the control model. The Kaiser model had no impact in the insulin-only group. 2. Among oral hypoglycemic users (with or without insulin), the Kaiser model was associated with a decrease in total costs of 21.9% per prescription filled as compared to the control model. The state model predicted a decrease in total costs of 9.9% per prescription filled as compared to the control model. **Limitations:** 1. Patients could go to any of the three pharmacy models to fill their prescriptions. Few patients used only one pharmacy, contaminating the intervention. 2. Self-selection into a particular pharmacy model may have been a problem. Two-stage least squares was used in an attempt to account for this, and results in the selection-corrected model differed from the uncorrected model.

Level of Focus	Reference	Setting/Population	Intervention	Results
System	Gerber & Stewart (1998)	**Setting:** West Baltimore, MD **Population:** Community-wide.	The intervention was based on the Baltimore Alliance for the Prevention and Control of Hypertension and Diabetes, a community-based program that includes the University of Maryland School of Medicine Center for Health Policy Research, the Joslin Diabetes Center, several MCO partners, Legacy 2000 (a Baltimore newspaper's men's health initiative), Millennium Healthcare (a health education and services organization), and a pharmaceutical company (Hoechst Marion Roussel). The program involves the use of community health workers and is modeled on the Barefoot Doctor program in China. Church-based education and screening works to enroll patients in treatment programs. The program is designed to mobilize the community in the management of hypertension and diabetes and to provide culturally relevant care. Care includes stepped, achievable goals that encourage patients to take control of their own disease management.	1. No assessment of intervention is reported. **Limitations:** 1. Only a description of intervention was provided.

Level of Focus	Reference	Setting/Population	Intervention	Results
System	Rubin et al. (1998)	**Setting:** Seven HMOs across the United States **Population:** Memberwide, implementation at seven HMOs nationwide, including more than 7,000 diabetic patients.	Diabetes NetCare is a comprehensive diabetes-management program designed by Diabetes Treatment Centers of America for implementation in managed care settings. NetCare provides external management of diabetic populations through intensive management of diabetes, designed to mimic care provided during the Diabetes Control and Complications Trial (DCCT). NetCare profiles an organization's diabetic population, costs and utilization and tailors a management program to the particular MCO. Management includes coordination of care among physicians, hospitals, and other care providers. In addition, NetCare stratifies the diabetic population into severity levels and focuses resources on the most severe cases. All patients are assigned to a diabetes case manager and are taught diabetes self-management skills. Patients with elevated HbA1c levels are assigned to complex-case managers who more intensely manage care. NetCare provides an on-site administrative team, a clinical team, a provider support team, a management team, and an electronic tracking system to each purchasing MCO.	1. The portion of patients with at least one HbA1c in the follow-up year rose from 34% to 76%. 2. Eye exam rates, foot exam rates, and cholesterol testing rates rose from 23% to 40%, from 2% to 25%, and from 39% to 63%, respectively. 3. Following the intervention, hospital admissions decreased from 239 per 1,000 diabetic member-years to 196 per 1,000 diabetic member-years. Bed days decreased from 1,336 during the baseline year to 1,047 in the intervention year. Average length of stay decreased from 5.6 days to 5.3 days. 4. Total costs decreased by 10.9% following the intervention, an average of $44 per diabetic member per month. The largest decrease in costs occurred because of decreased hospitalization costs. Nondiabetic patients experienced a 1.4% increase in costs during the same time period. 5. Physicians gave the program high ratings overall, whereas patients had a more tempered response. Limitations: 1. Follow-up was shorter than 12 months for five of the plans included. Accurate annual event counts are not possible (results may be understated). 2. QoL and satisfaction survey response rates were low.

Level of Focus	Reference	Setting/Population	Intervention	Results
System	Chicoye et al. (1998)	**Setting:** Primecare, a United Health Care company, the largest HMO network in Wisconsin **Population:** Memberwide, all patients with diabetes enrolled in the plan identified through claims data ($N = 5,100$).	The Diabetes Care Management program developed by Primecare was implemented. The initiative is described as a systemic approach to managing diabetes care; it includes practice guidelines, standards of care, patient education, mailed reminders to patients and physicians, and informal relationships with the ADA, local bureau of public health, and pharmaceutical companies.	1. The portion of patients receiving an HbA1c rose from 44% to 57% ($p < .01$). 2. Eye examination rates rose from 26% to 30% ($p < .01$). 3. Lipid-testing rates rose from 58% to 92%. **Limitations:** 1. Eye examination rates remained low after the intervention. 2. Results are from an informal evaluation. No formal study was conducted.
System	Friedman et al. (1996, 1998) Terry (1997)	**Setting:** Lovelace Health System, Albuquerque, NM **Population:** Memberwide, all diabetic patients within the Lovelace system.	Episodes of Care (EOC) disease-management program was developed for diabetic enrollees. A systematic method of disease management was developed to correct fragmented care processes in the health plan. EOC teams of caregivers were created to engage providers in clinical process improvement, including improvement of system performance, reduction of inappropriate care, reduction of costs, improvement of quality, and promotion of customer service. The program includes a patient-monitoring card that patients use to track their own care over the course of a year. The EOC program is available for sale to external organizations.	1. HbA1c levels in the patient population decreased from $12.2\% \pm 3.09$ in 1994 to $11.39\% \pm 2.92$ in 1995 ($p < .01$) to $10.4\% \pm 2.66$ in 1996 ($p < .005$). 2. The rate of annual dilated eye exams rose from 47.3% in 1994 to 53.2% in 1996. This was not considered to be a substantial improvement by the authors. 3. The portion of the population receiving diabetic education rose from 52% in 1993 to 78% in 1995. **Limitations:** Results reported are only for the HEDIS population, not for the enrolled patient population.

Level of Focus	Reference	Setting/Population	Intervention	Results
System	Gilmet et al. (1998)	**Setting:** Blue Care Network of Southeast Michigan, an HMO, independent licensee of Blue Cross/Blue Shield. **Population:** Memberwide, all plan enrollees identified as diabetic through claims.	Disease-management reports are generated from administrative claims and pharmacy data. The reports were used as behavior change and educational tools for physicians. Reports contained disease-, patient-, and physician-level data regarding diabetes management, focusing primarily on HbA1c levels. They were intended to provide physicians with feedback, aid decision making, promote adherence to guidelines, and measure outcomes improvement over time. The program was part of the Adult Diabetes Education Program and Training (ADEPT) taking place in the plan.	1. Results presented were simple counts of procedures ordered and the number of diabetics in the system. This information will be used to refine outcomes management. **Limitations:** 1. Only a description of disease-management intentions was provided. No implementation or evaluation of the interventions was described.

Level of Focus	Reference	Setting/Population	Intervention	Results
System	Ginsberg et al. (1998) Mazze et al. (1994)	**Setting:** Developed by the International Diabetes Center at multiple sites both in the United States and globally **Population:** Memberwide, implemented in multiple sites internationally.	Stage Diabetes Management (SDM) is a program for diabetes management developed by the International Diabetes Center and implemented in more than 100 international sites. The program emphasizes community involvement in care, aggressive treatment time lines set in cooperation with patients, the use of flowcharts in medical decision making and program evaluation. Windows-based care protocols link to clinical outcomes information and patient medical records.	1. Sites employing SDM were able to achieve reductions in HbA1c levels similar to those achieved during the DCCT (reduction of about 2%). 2. Preliminary cost information suggests that SDM cost about $1,500 per patient in the first year of implementation and $800 per patient per year in subsequent years. When savings from acute and chronic complications were factored into cost equations, the program broke even in terms of cost in 6 to 7 years. Lifetime savings from SDM were estimated to be $27,000 per patient (net present value). **Limitations:** 1. Results were not based on formal evaluations of SDM, but on discussions of general findings from implementation at multiple sites. 2. Cost estimates were not based on a formal cost-benefit analysis.
System	Heinen et al. (1993)	**Setting:** Multiple United HealthCare plans **Population:** Memberwide, implemented in 18 of United HealthCare's IPA-network plans.	Quality Screening Management (QSM) is a trademarked methodology developed by United HealthCare to identify areas for quality improvement in its IPA plans. QSM is used in United HealthCare's 18 managed care plans and is also available for purchase. Within disease categories (including diabetes, asthma), QSM compares plans to each other and to national practice guidelines, using claims data and medical record review. Simple quality-improvement actions are suggested by the QSM teams.	1. No results were reported. **Limitations:** 1. Only a description of the intervention was provided; no results were reported.

Level of Focus	Reference	Setting/Population	Intervention	Results
System	O'Connor et al. (1996) O'Connor & Pronk, (1998)	**Setting:** Two clinics at a staff model HMO in Minneapolis, MN (HealthPartners) **Population:** Memberwide, all diabetic patients enrolled in intervention clinic ($n = 134$) compared to diabetic population of a control clinic ($n = 133$).	A pilot version of Project IDEAL, a CQI initiative developed cooperatively between the Centers for Disease Control, the Minnesota Department of Health, and HealthPartners of Minneapolis was implemented at HealthPartners. The intervention is based on a 13-stage model of diabetes management, which includes scrutiny of current care processes, identification of barriers to quality care, development of alternative strategies, implementation of changes, and evaluation of results. The model is driven by staff implementation of changes in care. Protocols for patient education and patient care processes were developed.	1. In the intervention clinic, 78% of patients had at least one HbA1c in the first year of the program and 91% had at least one HbA1c in Year 2. In the control clinic, these proportions were 71% and 91% respectively. 2. Of those with an HbA1c test, good control was observed in 51% of intervention clinic patients versus 40% of control clinic patients; poor control was observed in 12% of intervention clinic patients versus 27% of control clinic patients. Glycemic control was judged to be significantly better in the intervention clinic than in the control clinic. 3. During Year 1, average HbA1c levels were slightly higher in the control clinic as compared to the intervention clinic (8.4% versus 8.9%, $p < .06$). During Years 2 and 3, average HbA1c in the control clinic was significantly higher than in the intervention clinic (8.9% versus 8.0%, $p < .001$ in Year 2; 8.8% versus 7.9%, $p < .001$ in Year 3). 4. Controlling for baseline HbA1c, intervention-group patients had a significantly greater decrease in HbA1c compared to controls. 5. The mean number of outpatient visits increased in both groups. 6. Outpatient costs in the control clinic increased by 29% compared to a 27% increase in the intervention clinic. This does not include the cost of the intervention. Limitations: 1. Mean HbA1c levels in both clinics started so near to the normal range that it would be difficult to observe large decreases in these levels.

Level of Focus	Reference	Setting/Population	Intervention	Results
System	Solberg et al. (1997)	**Setting:** Three HealthPartners clinics in Minneapolis, MN, involved in 1996 pilot. Randomized controlled trial scheduled to begin in 13 HealthPartners clinics in 1997. **Population:** Memberwide description of intervention only, no population used for evaluation.	The IDEAL (Improving Care for Diabetes through Empowerment, Active Collaboration and Leadership) program was developed by HealthPartners of Minnesota. IDEAL is a CQI approach used by HealthPartners to improve diabetes care through its primary-care clinics. HealthPartners has worked collaboratively with the Centers for Disease Control on this initiative. The IDEAL program consisted of three interconnected processes: the intervention process, the improvement process and the care delivery process. This systematic approach to care was intended to reduce variations in care and routinize comprehensive care for diabetic patients.	1. No results were presented. **Limitations:** 1. There was only a description of the IDEAL model; no evaluation results were presented.
System	Wagner (1995)	**Setting:** Group Health Cooperative of Puget Sound (systemwide) **Population:** Memberwide description of intervention only, no population used for evaluation.	Population-based disease management was implemented for all diabetic patients enrolled in Group Health Cooperative of Puget Sound. This approach consists of six components: (a) identification of the diabetic population enrolled, (b) definition of relevant changeable outcomes, (c) development of clinical guidelines based on ADA recommendations, (d) selection and implementation of interventions known to be effective, (e) monitoring performance and outcomes, and (f) altering delivery approach. The care system adopted a model of miniclinics, devoting blocks of time to diabetic patients, and adopted a clinical computing system to track adherence with guidelines. Implementation of effective interventions involved the identification of barriers to care delivery.	1. No results were reported. **Limitations:** 1. There was only a description of the intervention; no evaluation results were presented.

Level of Focus	Reference	Setting/Population	Intervention	Results
System	Joshi & Bernard (1999)	**Setting:** University of Pennsylvania Health System **Population:** Memberwide: Diabetic patients at all practice sites in the system were affected by the intervention.	A CQI initiative was implemented through the leadership of a multidisciplinary management team. The initiative was based on using best-practice guidelines to provide care to diabetic patients. Elements of the program included diabetes case managers providing care to high-risk patients, multidisciplinary care teams, use of clinical practice guidelines, health risk assessment, and stratification of patients by disease severity. Nurse case managers focused on care for high-risk patients but also contacted low-risk patients periodically by phone. Case managers worked closely with physicians. Physicians from each of the system's clinic sites joined planning meetings to smooth the introduction of the initiative into their clinic sites.	1. Patients reported a high level of satisfaction with the program. 2. The system is currently developing a strategy for assessing the financial viability of the program. **Limitations:** 1. The article describes the CQI initiatives for multiple conditions taking place in the health system. The description of the diabetes initiative itself is limited. No results of formal evaluation of the diabetes initiative are reported.

Appendix B: Literature Describing Asthma Management Programs in Managed Care Organizations

Level of Focus	Reference	Setting/Population	Intervention	Results
Patient	Kowal (1997)	**Setting:** Blue Cross/Blue Shield of Massachusetts **Population:** Memberwide: Program is intended to affect all asthmatic members of the MCO.	The Adult Outpatient Asthma Education Project has two primary goals: (a) increase patient education and (b) increase inhaled anti-inflammatory use. The program includes staff education weekly and one-on-one education sessions with a nurse educator. The nurse receives a daily list of patients seen in the emergency room or hospitalized for asthma. The nurse identifies barriers to asthma care and identifies patients who need education. Patients with complex asthma are scheduled for appointments with a pulmonologist. Letters are sent to patients' primary-care providers regarding the use of anti-inflammatory inhalers among patients who are eligible candidates for their use. Letters also are sent to primary-care physicians regarding patients who fill bronchodilator prescriptions more than once per month.	1. The author reports that consultations with asthma specialists resulted in reduced hospitalizations and emergency-room visits. 2. The use of anti-inflammatory inhalers among eligible patients increased from 30% to 60% over 2 years. 3. A 50% decrease in costs among asthma patients was observed after 1 year, accompanied by a 40% decrease in hospital admissions. **Limitations:** 1. The results presented are brief, study population is not described, and a method of cost calculation is not described.

Level of Focus	Reference	Setting/Population	Intervention	Results
Patient	Wilson-Pessano et al. (1987) Wilson et al. (1993)	**Setting:** Five Kaiser Permanente Northern California plans **Population:** Programwide: All plan enrollees treated for asthma in a 6-month period prior to intervention or seen in the emergency room for asthma were randomized into educational interventions or control groups ($N = 570$).	Randomized controlled trial was conducted of the AIRWISE and AIRPOWER asthma educational programs adapted for adults. Patients were randomized into one of two educational programs (AIRWISE or AIRPOWER), an attention/information control, or a data-only control. The AIRWISE program involved one-on-one education focused on medication management. AIRPOWER used group education sessions. Both programs emphasized a set of core competencies in the following areas: (a) effective use of medical, educational, and interpersonal resources; (b) symptoms management; (c) use of medications to prevent symptoms; (d) avoidance of triggers; and (e) maintenance of general physical and mental well-being. Both programs involved four to five weekly sessions. Both programs emphasized self-monitoring, goal-setting, and behavioral contracting.	1. Patients in educational groups demonstrated greater knowledge regarding medications than patients in control groups. 2. Rates of hospitalization between educational groups and control groups did not differ. 3. At 5 months, patients in the education groups had significantly lower "bother from asthma" ratings and significantly fewer symptom days, but these differences did not persist after 5 months. 4. Educational groups demonstrated more improvement in asthma as assessed by a physician when compared to controls. Patients receiving different types of education did not differ from each other. 5. Education-group patients reported higher levels of activity than control-group patients. 6. Participation in an educational group was associated with reduced acute office visits in the second 12 months following the intervention but not for the first 12 months or for the entire study period. A reduction in acute office visits in this population was not accompanied by an increase in scheduled office visits. **Limitations:** 1. Results are somewhat ambiguous. The educational program seems best at improving knowledge about asthma but does not seem to make a measurable difference in health outcomes. 2. Patients deemed eligible for study were significantly more compliant with medication regimens (as rated by their physicians) than patients who were excluded from the study.

Level of Focus	Reference	Setting/Population	Intervention	Results
Patient	Forshee et al. (1998)	**Setting:** Four predominantly IPA-model plans: Mid Atlantic Medical Services Inc. (Rockville, MD), Blue Cross and Blue Shield of Western New York (Buffalo, NY), Blue Cross and Blue Shield of Kansas City, and Blue Care Network of East Michigan (Saginaw, MI) **Population:** Programwide: Adult and child asthma patients identified as being at high-risk were enrolled (N = 280).	A nurse-led education program for high-risk adult and pediatric asthma patients from four managed care plans was implemented. Nurse champions, trained in asthma patient management, organized patient education either at patients' homes or at clinics. Nurses were trained using the INSPIRE program developed by Integrated Therapeutics Group. The basic patient-contact program consisted of one baseline visit and four follow-up contacts by the nurse champion every 6 weeks. Patients were trained in medications, treatment guidelines, warning signs, and use of peak-flow meters (PFMs). The first two follow-up contacts with patients were by phone. The second two contacts took place at the patient's home.	1. Patients demonstrated improvement in asthma knowledge, which was sustained over the intervention period (24 weeks). Patients demonstrated significant improvement in their knowledge of how to treat a flare-up. 2. Patients and patient caregivers demonstrated improved confidence in their ability to care for asthma. 3. There was a significant increase in the number of patients using inhaled anti-inflammatory medications. 4. There was a significant increase in the proportion of patients referred to specialists for care. 5. Significant decreases in asthma severity (as classified by the nurse champion) were observed for adults and children. The improvements were sustained throughout the intervention. 6. The intervention was associated with improvements in QoL for both adult asthma patients and for caregivers of child patients. 7. Significant decreases in urgent care, emergency-room visits, and hospitalizations were observed in the population. The monthly rate of outpatient visits increased significantly in the population. **Limitations:** 1. 30% of patients were lost to follow-up. Enrollment from each plan was small, ranging from 22 to 65 patients. 2. The follow-up period was short (24 weeks).

Level of Focus	Reference	Setting/Population	Intervention	Results
Patient	Wilson et al. (1996)	**Setting:** Two sites: Aspen Medical Group (St. Paul, MN) and St. Paul Children's Hospital (St. Paul, MN) **Population:** Programwide: Patients continuously enrolled who had three or more asthma visits in the previous year were recruited and randomized to treatment and control groups ($N = 76$).	The Wee Wheezers asthma educational program was designed for parents of children with asthma who were under 7 years old. The program consists of four 2-hour small-group sessions that cover prevention of symptoms; management of symptoms; use of medical, educational, and social resources; communication with adults responsible for the child's care; and promotion of the psychological well-being of the family. Children ages 4 to 6 received instruction at the same time as their parents and were taught how to use PFMs and metered dose inhalers (MDIs) and how to recognize symptoms. Children under 4 received no direct instruction. The program included the development of a written asthma action plan tailored for each child and booster sessions at 3 and 6 months after initial intervention.	1. About 95% of intervention-group parents attended at least three of the four educational sessions. 2. The control group had a significantly greater increase in symptom days and nights of interrupted parental sleep compared to the intervention group (increases occurred in both groups.) 3. The intervention group had an increase in symptom-free days, whereas the control experienced a decrease; the difference between them was statistically significant. 4. The groups did not differ in the change in "asthma bother" ratings over the preceding 3 months or in sick days. **Limitations:** 1. There is the potential for volunteer bias: Of 129 people originally invited to participate, more than 50 refused to participate.

Level of Focus	Reference	Setting/Population	Intervention	Results
Patient	Griffin et al. (1989) Shields et al. (1990)	**Setting:** Two inner-city health care centers of an urban HMO in Chicago. **Population:** Programwide: children with recent emergency-room use randomized into usual care or intervention group (N = 253).	An educational program was implemented for inner-city children. The program consisted of small-group classes for parents and children and telephone contact by a nurse clinician. The educational objective included 23 skill mastery areas in four main categories: prevention of attacks, medication management, intervention during attacks, and utilization of resources. Only 38% of the intervention group participated in one or more of the four classes offered, so primary contact was made through telephone in many cases. Frequency of phone contact depended on severity of illness, but all parents were contacted at least once per season. Phone calls lasted about 30 minutes.	1. After 1 year, there were no differences between intervention and control groups in use of health care services, emergency-room use, hospitalization, or outpatient use. 2. The intervention was thought to have failed because of inadequate focus on motivating behavior change. The authors felt that the program failed because it was not tailored to suit a low-income minority population. 3. The study did not assess changes in functional status or sick days and focused primarily on measures of service utilization. **Limitations:** 1. Primarily, contacts were made by phone rather than through the planned intervention because of low attendance at educational sessions. Ultimately, the study does not represent an evaluation of the planned intervention because attendance was so low.
Patient	Moe et al. (1992)	**Setting:** Kaiser Permanente Northwest region (Portland, OR). **Population:** Programwide, children referred by primary-care physician, identified by emergency-room use and afterhours care use or by pharmacy records (N = 74).	The Open Airways program, adapted for a nonminority, non-inner city population, was implemented. Parents and children attended separate education sessions that focused on asthma triggers, medications, and management of physical activity and problems in school. Families discussed goal setting and development of a written plan of action for managing child asthma. Children's education includes puppet shows, activities, and practice with inhalers. Phone and mail follow-up occurred if a family missed a training session.	1. About 84% of enrolled families attended at least one class; 32% attended all six classes. Of those who attended at least one session, 79% attended at least five sessions. 2. Parental confidence in taking care of child asthma increased significantly. **Limitations:** 1. This was essentially a descriptive study of the program and its adaptation for a non-Hispanic population. No formal evaluation was conducted. No results of the program's impact on health outcomes or utilization were reported.

Level of Focus	Reference	Setting/Population	Intervention	Results
Patient	McNabb et al. (1985)	**Setting:** Patients were recruited from the allergy clinics of multiple Kaiser Permanente Northern California clinics. **Population:** Programwide: Children with at least one emergency-room visit for asthma within the previous year were recruited. Intervention group compared to controls ($N = 14$).	AIR WISE, an asthma education program for children, was used. The program included four weekly, 1-hour, one-on-one education sessions for children with asthma and their parents. The self-management problems for each child were assessed and the educational program tailored to meet individual needs. AIR WISE uses goal setting, self-evaluation, and self-monitoring to encourage behavior change.	1. In the 12 months following the intervention, the intervention group averaged 1.9 emergency-room visits, and the control group averaged 7.4 emergency-room visits. Prior to the intervention, average emergency-room visits were 6.1 per 12 months among intervention-group patients and 5.7 per 12 months among control-group patients. 2. There was no difference between groups in non-emergency room visits or drug usage. 3. The authors reported improvement among the intervention group members in knowledge about asthma and self-management behaviors. **Limitations:** 1. The sample size was extremely small. This group was divided into a control and treatment group. It is impossible to conduct statistical testing or infer generalizability given the small sample size.

Level of Focus	Reference	Setting/Population	Intervention	Results
Patient	Lewis et al. (1984)*	**Setting:** Kaiser Permanente Sunset Clinic and West Los Angeles Clinic in Los Angeles **Population:** Programwide: Patients with severe asthma, between 7 and 12 years of age, and fluent in English were selected. Intervention group compared to control group ($N = 76$).	Asthma Care Training (ACT) for Kids was tested in a randomized controlled trial. Intervention-group patients and families were enrolled in ACT, which included five weekly 1-hour education sessions with parents and children separated for 45 minutes and joined together for a 15-minute wrap-up session. The program for children included education through games, simulation, and modeling. The curriculum was designed by nurses, health educators, and elementary school teachers. The program emphasizes children taking control of their asthma. Control-group patients and families attended three 1-hour educational sessions covering the same information as the intervention group.	1. The intervention had a significant impact on the number of emergency-room visits and an impact of borderline significance on the number of hospitalizations. The intervention group had a statistically significant decrease in hospitalization days, whereas hospitalization days among the control group increased. 2. The authors estimated a net savings from the program of $180 per child per year (1984 dollars). 3. Both groups demonstrated a significant decrease in perceived severity of episodes. Both groups of parents rated their children's health status as significantly improved at 1 year postintervention. 4. Improvements in self-management behaviors were reported among both groups. **Limitations:** 1. Children were required to be fluent in English. It is unclear whether parents were also required to be English speakers. Such a requirement could exclude Hispanic patients served by the clinics. 2. The authors report that program dropouts were overwhelmingly Latino and black.

*Despite the fact that this article does not fall within the parameters of the data range selected for this review (1985-1999), we have included it because it is a widely recognized and important reference in the area of asthma programs.

Level of Focus	Reference	Setting/Population	Intervention	Results
Provider	Buchner et al. (1998)	**Setting:** Atlantic Medical Services, Inc., an IPA-network HMO **Population:** Memberwide, asthmatic members identified through claims entered in program ($N = 6,698$).	This is a disease-management intervention cooperatively implemented by an IPA, Integrated Therapeutics Group (ITG, a subsidiary of Schering-Plough), and Diversified Pharmaceutical Services (DPS, a PBM). Physicians were trained in NHLBI guidelines for asthma care and provided with asthma kits by ITG to give to their patients. DPS identified asthmatic patients through administrative claims and provided physicians with profiles of their patients' medication use. Patients identified through claims were offered asthma-education classes coordinated by ITG.	1. The number of prescriptions for inhaled corticosteroids increased by 30%, and the proportion of asthmatics on chronic therapy increased by 25%. 2. The use of inpatient services in the population decreased by 18%. The proportion of asthmatics with multiple hospitalizations decreased significantly. 3. The proportion of patients with one or more visits to the emergency room remained unchanged. 4. General health status did not change among adults, but improvement on disease-specific health-related QoL scales was reported. Children's health status (as reported by parents) improved for both general and disease-specific measures. 5. No change in patients' satisfaction with their health plan was reported. **Limitations:** 1. No information was provided on the decrease in hospitalization rates that occurred for the health system as a whole. 2. No evidence of a sustained impact of this intervention was provided.

Level of Focus	Reference	Setting/Population	Intervention	Results
Provider	Plaut et al. (1996)	**Setting:** Principle Health Care of Louisiana (IPA-network HMO), member of a national MCO (Principle Health Care) **Population:** Memberwide: Target population for Year 1 was asthmatic children; adults were added in Year 2.	The HMO implemented a primary care-provider education project designed by consultant Thomas Plaut. The intervention was designed to support primary-care providers in their care of asthma patients by providing them with education regarding guidelines, early diagnosis, use of medications, preventive treatment, and monitoring of patients. Three pediatricians, an internist, and two allergists were selected to act as liaisons between the health care plan and providers who care for asthma patients. A nurse/case manager was used to oversee patient and family support networks. The program included home-care visits for patient education and use of patient-education materials authored by Plaut. The program included a series of conferences conducted by Plaut for physicians, nurses, respiratory therapists, local school nurses, and other clinic staff. The program was designed for a 2-year implementation, beginning with children as the target population. After 1 year, adult asthmatics were added to the program.	1. No results presented. **Limitations:** 1. This article is a description of the program only. No outcomes results were reported.

Level of Focus	Reference	Setting/Population	Intervention	Results
System	Zeiger et al. (1991)	**Setting:** Kaiser Health Plan HMO, San Diego **Population:** Programwide, enrollees with emergency-room visit or hospitalization for asthma in 1988 randomized to treatment or control group ($N = 309$).	The article describes a prospective, randomized, controlled trial of referral to asthma-care specialists. Patients in the intervention group received an expedited allergy-clinic evaluation and were followed by allergists and asthma-care specialists. Patients received education regarding medications, environmental triggers, and PFM use. The use of inhaled anti-inflammatory agents was emphasized in intervention group. The control group received routine care from generalists.	1. The intervention group exhibited significantly better asthma control after 6 months than the control group (as measured on a 5-point scale). 2. A greater proportion of the intervention group as compared to the control group used inhaled corticosteroids or inhaled cromolyn after 6 months. Oral medications were used at similar rates in both groups. 3. In multivariate analysis, membership in the intervention group was significantly associated with reduced emergency-room relapses. **Limitations:** 1. Outcomes were measured at 6 months (a relatively short time horizon.)
System	Greineder et al. (1995)	**Setting:** Harvard Community Health Plan's Kenmore Center (staff-model HMO in Boston). Clinic population is predominantly low socioeconomic status. **Population:** Programwide, patients with emergency-room visits and hospitalizations identified; high-risk patients also referred by physicians ($N = 53$).	A nurse-coordinated outreach clinic was developed to help draw patients in an urban area into a pediatric asthma-education program. The clinic was staffed by two nurse practitioners who had access to an allergist for consultation. Children and their families received 2 hours of one-on-one education in which asthma triggers and medications were reviewed and an asthma control program was developed. A second visit was scheduled if necessary, and families received weekly telephone follow-up from the nurse. The nurse reviewed medications with the allergist or physician if a problem was suspected.	1. Emergency-room visits and hospitalizations in the 12 months following the intervention were significantly lower than in the 12 months prior to intervention. **Limitations:** 1. The sample size was small.

Level of Focus	Reference	Setting/Population	Intervention	Results
System	Greineder et al. (1999)	**Setting:** Harvard Community Health Plan, patients drawn from multiple urban clinics **Population:** Programwide: pediatric patients recruited from hospitalization lists; high-risk patients also referred by physicians. Patients compared to a randomized group of controls ($N = 89$).	Asthma Outreach Program (AOP) for children is a more fully developed version of a previous nurse-coordinated outreach clinic at Harvard Community Health Plan. A one-on-one education program was scheduled with patient and family in which a written asthma-control plan was developed, use of MDI and PFM was reviewed, and referral to an allergist was made if allergies were thought to be present. Program design was based on NHLBI guidelines. Control group patients received education only, with no long-term follow-up.	1. Emergency-room use and hospitalizations declined significantly in both the control and intervention groups 1 year after the intervention. 2. Outside-of-plan use was also significantly less in both groups following intervention. 3. Reductions in emergency-room use, hospitalization, and outside-of-plan use were significantly larger in the intervention group compared to the control group. 4. For patients in the intervention group, $11.67 was saved for every $1 invested in the outreach nurse who coordinated the program. **Limitations:** 1. The sample size was small.
System	Kropfelder (1996)	**Setting:** Kaiser Permanente Baltimore **Population:** Programwide: Patients with emergency-room visits or hospitalizations in the year prior to the intervention ($N = 114$).	A nurse case-management program was developed for pediatric patients and their parents. The inner-city patient population generally had a difficult time returning to their clinics for education and appointments, so the program was geared toward phone contact with patients. Families who were able attended education classes. A written asthma-care program based on guidelines and peak-flow measurement was developed for each family, with its primary-care physician. Phone contact was made with patients in days prior to clinic appointments.	1. In the first year of the program, emergency-room visits declined by 50%, and hospitalizations declined by 66%. 2. These reductions were accompanied by a 25% increase in outpatient visits. **Limitations:** 1. No formal evaluation of the program was conducted. Results were presented briefly and informally.

Level of Focus	Reference	Setting/Population	Intervention	Results
System	Stevens & Weiss-Harrison (1993)	**Setting:** Kaiser-Permanente, White Plains, NY **Population:** Memberwide, all patients who sought care in the clinic.	The program involved a nurse home-visit intervention for pediatric asthma patients, developed by consultant Thomas Plaut. The primary goal of the program was to reduce hospitalizations for asthmatics under age 15. Nurses delivered nebulizers and PFMs to patients and taught patients proper use during home visits. Equipment was provided to patients at no cost. Education on medication use continued at regular office visits. Pediatricians and nurse practitioners worked together to develop a management strategy for patients on a case-by-case basis.	1. Hospitalization days showed a downward trend for the years following the intervention. **Limitations:** 1. There was no formal evaluation of the intervention.

Level of Focus	Reference	Setting/Population	Intervention	Results
System	Trubitt (1999)	**Setting:** United HealthCare of Illinois **Population:** Programwide: Program is targeted toward pediatric patients with high numbers of hospitalizations or high asthma-care costs ($N = 250$ initially identified for the program).	A multifaceted intervention was implemented to improve health outcomes for high-risk asthmatic enrollees. Intervention elements included improved access to specialist care, increased communication between primary-care providers and asthma-care specialists through the use of a hot line, and designation of three hospitals as asthma-care centers.	1. The investigators had difficulty keeping patients enrolled in the program. One third of the enrolled patients simply did not keep appointments and were eventually dropped from the study. Two thirds of the patient population were Medicaid enrollees, and many lost their Medicaid eligibility during the course of the program evaluation. Many enrollees did not have telephones and could not be reached for appointment scheduling and follow-up. 2. Among those patients for whom data were available ($n = 88$), the authors report reductions in inpatient days and inpatient costs. 3. Among those patients for whom QoL data were available ($n = 57$), the authors note improvements in symptom-free days, school days lost, and sleep lost. **Limitations:** 1. This article provides only a brief description of the intervention and results. A formal description and evaluation of the program was in press at the time information for this volume was collected. 2. The potential success of this intervention is hampered by extremely high dropout rates in the population. Results are based on limited subsets of the enrolled population.

Level of Focus	Reference	Setting/Population	Intervention	Results
System	Goonan et al. (1993)	**Setting:** Harvard Community Health Plan **Population:** Memberwide, program focused on all asthmatic children in the plan.	A CQI initiative involving strategic planning for the care of all enrolled asthmatic children was implemented. The program involved creation of a multidisciplinary team charged with implementing disease-management initiatives. Patient needs assessment was conducted by survey and focus groups. The impact of an asthma-outreach nurse was investigated in a pilot study. An electronic medical records system was developed to improve availability of medical records to clinicians treating asthma patients.	1. No results were presented. **Limitations:** 1. The article is a description of a disease-management strategy and tools for assessment and benchmarking. No results or analysis of impact were presented.
System	Terry (1997)	**Setting:** Lovelace Health System, Albuquerque, NM **Population:** Memberwide, all enrollees in the health system.	Lovelace Health System has developed an Episodes of Care (EOC) disease management strategy. An EOC is defined as all of the services provided to a patient with a particular medical problem within a defined time period. In the case of a chronic condition like asthma, an episode represents a lifetime of care. Asthma as an episode has an EOC team that includes specialists, primary-care physicians, nurse care managers, education specialists, and quality measurement specialists. The EOC team is responsible for developing care protocols and practice guidelines for the target episode. The goal of the EOC method is to reduce inappropriate care, improve system performance, and improve customer satisfaction.	1. A 34% reduction in hospitalizations for pediatric asthma was reported. **Limitations:** 1. This article is not a formal evaluation of the EOC interventions and contains information about interventions for several conditions.

Level of Focus	Reference	Setting/Population	Intervention	Results
System	Ellenbecker et al. (1998)	**Setting:** More than 80 hospitals that deliver care to Medicaid patients in Massachusetts. **Population:** Memberwide: All hospitals in Massachusetts serving Medicaid beneficiaries participated.	The Asthma Education and Primary Care Clinician Linkages Quality Improvement Project (QIP) is one part of the ongoing Hospital Quality Initiative in Massachusetts. All hospitals serving Medicaid patients in the state were mandated to work toward achieving two goals: (a) provide and document patient education to all Medicaid beneficiaries hospitalized or seen in the emergency room for asthma and (b) establish a written or verbal communication system with patient's primary-care provider that includes notification of patient stay in the emergency room or hospital and notification of any follow-up care delivered. Hospitals were required to submit patient-education materials, asthma-care protocols or guidelines, and documentation of facilitated communication with primary-care providers.	1. Most hospitals were in the process of developing a QIP program at the request of the state, not by their own initiative. 2. More than half of the reporting hospitals used practice guidelines for the care of asthma. 3. Most hospitals had asthma educational materials, but only 32% had a plan for dissemination of the materials, and only 49% could name a person responsible for asthma education. 4. The majority of hospitals did not have a plan in place for communicating with primary-care providers of asthma patients, and 31% of hospitals had no intention of developing such a plan. **Limitations:** 1. This study examined results of QIP's request for submission from more than 80 contracting hospitals regarding their asthma-care programs and supporting data. There was no discussion of the impact of QIP on health outcomes for asthma patients.

Level of Focus	Reference	Setting/Population	Intervention	Results
System	Wilson et al. (1998)	**Setting:** Fresno, CA **Population:** Community-wide, intervention targeted at the entire Fresno County, California, population.	The Fresno Asthma Project (FAP) was a cooperative effort undertaken by the American Institutes of Research (AIR), the local American Lung Association, Kaiser Permanente, and the San Joaquin Valley Health Consortium. The intervention was focused on improving asthma morbidity and mortality among the multiethnic, low-income population of the area. The FAP consists of three components: professional education, patient education, and community education. Guidelines-based educational programs for professionals (including physicians, community health providers, teachers, and day care providers) and patients were developed by Kaiser Permanente and AIR. Educational programs were offered at Kaiser clinic sites, as well as in schools and at work sites. Educational programs were translated into Spanish and Hmong.	1. Following implementation of the program, MCOs operating in the area began to sponsor their own asthma-education programs. The authors suggest that increased involvement by MCOs occurred because of the successful impact of the programs offered by the FAP. **Limitations:** 1. The article contained only a description of the FAP. No evaluation of the impact of the intervention on health outcomes in the population was provided.

Level of Focus	Reference	Setting/Population	Intervention	Results
System	Ludwig-Beymer & Greene (1999)	**Setting:** Advocate Health Care, a nonprofit integrated delivery system including eight hospitals in Chicago **Population:** Memberwide: All patients seeking care within the Advocate system are affected by the program.	The development of the Adult Asthma Program began with the identification of hospitalization rates among adults using system hospitals. The extent of emergency-department and hospital utilization were determined for each hospital in the system, and system physicians were surveyed about their asthma-care practices. An Adult Asthma Clinical Improvement Team was established to develop guidelines-based care protocols for various care settings, including the emergency room, hospital, and outpatient settings. Patient-education materials and a wallet card were also developed for patients. Patient-care flow sheets and an asthma classification scale were developed for outpatient providers. Partnerships with pharmaceutical companies were established by Advocate Health Care for the provision of educational materials and asthma-care supplies.	1. The authors report provider satisfaction with the materials provided. Some providers reported concern over the extra time required to follow protocols. **Limitations:** 1. The article presents primarily an informal description of the program. No formal evaluation of the program's impact is provided.

Appendix C: Literature Describing Congestive Heart Failure Management Programs in Managed Care Organizations

Non-Hospital Based Interventions

Level of Focus	Reference	Setting/Population	Intervention	Results
System	Brass-Mynderse (1996)	**Setting:** Scripps Health Chronic Care Clinic (La Jolla, CA) **Population:** Programwide, description of intervention only, no population used for evaluation. Any patient admitted to the affiliated hospital with CHF is eligible for the program.	This article describes a nurse-managed CHF clinic that serves patients on a risk-capitated basis. Advanced practice nurses and clinical specialist nurses follow treatment guidelines that have been integrated into a disease-management computer software program. Each patient was assigned an advanced practice nurse as his/her primary care provider. The clinic offered a 24-hour on-call nurse and a home health care specialty team. Patients were seen by a nurse weekly for the first 6 weeks after hospital release and monthly thereafter. Nurses focused on medication and dietary and lipid management with patients, as well as on exercise training, counseling, and other forms of patient education.	1. No results are presented. **Limitations:** 1. This was a description of an intervention only. No evaluation of the program was presented.

Level of Focus	Reference	Setting/Population	Intervention	Results
System	West et al. (1997)	**Setting:** Kaiser Permanente Medical Center, Hayward, CA **Population:** Programwide: Of 291 patients hospitalized during a specified time period, 238 were excluded from the study for various reasons. (Final study population $N = 51$.)	MULTIFIT is a nurse-managed, physician-supervised, home-based management program for CHF patients. Patient care was based on AHCPR, American College of Cardiology, and American Heart Association guidelines. Nurse case managers educated patients on disease state, diet, drug regimens, compliance, and symptoms in an initial visit. Patients' self-efficacy was assessed, and education was tailored to individual needs. Telephone contact with patients was maintained weekly for 6 weeks for symptom and medication monitoring. The 6-week telephone contact period was repeated if the patient experienced an emergency-room visit or hospitalization during the period. Worsening condition triggered increased phone contact. Patients whose disease remained stable received phone contact every 2 to 4 weeks for an additional 18 weeks. The program emphasized ACE-inhibitor use and monitoring of sodium intake.	1. In comparison with the 6 months prior to the intervention, 6-month rates for general medical visits declined 23% ($p < .03$), cardiology visits declined 31% ($p < .02$), emergency-room visits for CHF declined 67% ($p < .001$), and total emergency-room visits declined 53% ($p < .001$). 2. Compared to the 12 months prior to the intervention, CHF hospitalization rates declined 87% ($p < .0001$), and total hospitalizations declined 74% ($p < .0001$) in the 12 months following the intervention. 3. The proportion of patients with NYHA Class I or II compared to Class III or IV improved significantly at 3 and 6 months following implementation of the intervention. 4. Scores on the Duke Activity Status Index and on the physical component of the SF-36 improved significantly at 6 months. 5. Reported symptoms that significantly declined in severity after 6 months: cough, dyspnea on exertion, orthopnea, and fatigue. **Limitations:** 1. Results were based on a small sample size, particularly considering the number of hospitalized CHF patients who were considered ineligible for the program. This raises the issue of selection into the program of highly motivated patients.

Level of Focus	Reference	Setting/Population	Intervention	Results
System	Wilkes et al. (1999)	**Setting:** Kaiser Permanente South San Francisco (a staff-model HMO) **Population:** Programwide: From all enrolled CHF patients identified through claims information, high-risk patients (those with emergency-room visit or hospitalization) with left ventricular systolic dysfunction (LVSD) were targeted for intervention (N = 252).	The comprehensive management program that was implemented had three components: (a) CHF clinical pathway, (b) patient education module, and (c) case management. Prior to hospital discharge, nutritional, pharmacy, social, and physical therapy services consulted on the patient's care. Patients received at least one home health visit and were contacted by a case manager within 5 days of any hospitalization. The case manager arranged outpatient visits and provided follow-up phone calls. Patients attended outpatient classes consisting of five 2-hour sessions and received an educational manual. The program emphasized increased use of ACE inhibitors.	1. Hospital admissions for case-managed patients decreased by 22.7% over 18 months. 2. Average length of stay among case-managed patients decreased 12.8% over a 3-year period. Emergency-room visits in the population decreased by 21.7% over the same time period. 3. The CHF readmission rate within 5 days of discharge fell from 7.5 per 100 discharges to 3.0 per 100 discharges over a 3-year period in the study population. This represented the lowest readmission rate among CHF patients in the Kaiser Northern California system at that time. 4. ACE-inhibitor use among case-managed patients rose to 93% during the evaluation period. Limitations: 1. Statistical testing was not conducted. 2. Varying time periods were used for each outcome variable.

Hospital-Based Interventions

Level of Focus	Reference	Setting/Population	Intervention	Results
Patient	Clark et al. (1992)	**Setting:** Two large teaching hospitals **Population:** Programwide, older men and women randomly assigned to treatment and control groups ($N = 324$).	A patient-education program that consisted of a 2-hour group-education session for 8 to 10 adults per group held weekly for 4 weeks. The education program was based on social cognitive theory. Patients were taught problem recognition and problem solving through instruction, videotapes, and workbooks. Patients were taught to identify behavioral goals, develop a plan to achieve these goals, and devise a reward system for themselves. Topics covered included diet, medications, exercise, emotional well-being, rest, smoking, social relationships, communication with providers, and family interaction. Education sessions took place at the hospital.	1. At 12 months postintervention, the treatment group displayed significantly better QoL scores on the psychosocial, emotional, and alertness dimensions of the test. 2. Women in the treatment group had significantly better psychosocial scores and scores for work success than women in the control group. Women in the treatment group also had significantly better alertness scores than women in the control group. 3. Differences between men in the treatment group and men in the control group in psychosocial scores did not reach statistical significance. Men in the treatment group experienced significantly improved scores on the ambulation scale compared to men in the control group. **Limitations:** 1. Volunteer bias may have overstated positive results. The fairly intensive intervention attracted motivated subjects. 2. Reporting of dropouts was incomplete.

Level of Focus	Reference	Setting/Population	Intervention	Results
System	Rich et al. (1993)	**Setting:** Jewish Hospital at Washington University Medical Center (Missouri) **Population:** Programmwide: Intervention-group patients were compared with controls ($N = 98$). All patients 70 years or older and at high risk for readmission were entered into the study	A multidisciplinary intervention was designed to reduce hospital readmission rates. The intervention includes patient education from a geriatric cardiac nurse, a detailed review of medications by a geriatric cardiologist, dietary instruction, and discharge planning consultation with social services. The program also includes a home-care component. Patients receive home care within 48 hours of hospital discharge, receive home visits three times within the first week after discharge, and receive home visits and phone calls at regular intervals after the first week.	1. The readmission rate, time to readmission, and number of hospital days were not significantly different in the treatment and control groups following intervention, except in the high-risk group, in which intervention-group patients were more likely to be readmitted sooner than control-group patients ($p < .026$). Follow-up was for 90 days. 2. No significant trends toward lower rates of hospitalization and fewer hospitalization days appeared for the intervention-group patients classified as moderate risk patients. **Limitations:** 1. A large number of patients (or their physicians) refused to participate in the intervention or were excluded for other reasons that were not clearly explained. 2. There was a relatively short follow-up period.

Level of Focus	Reference	Setting/Population	Intervention	Results
System	Rich et al. (1995) Rich et al. (1996)	**Setting:** Jewish Hospital at Washington University Medical Center (Missouri) **Population:** Programwide, intervention group compared with controls ($N = 282$). All patients were 70 years or older. Patients at high risk for early readmission were excluded. Several other exclusion criteria applied.	This multidisciplinary intervention was intended to reduce hospital admissions (same as described in Rich et al. (1993), above, with further refinements). Patient education was conducted using a specially designed educational booklet. Patients received medication management, dietary instruction, discharge planning, and home care as described above.	1. Significantly more patients in the control group had at least one hospital readmission compared to intervention-group patients. Multiple readmissions were also significantly more prevalent in the control group as compared to the intervention group. Control-group patients also had significantly more total hospital days than treatment-group patients. 2. Treatment-group status was a significant predictor of readmission in multivariate analysis, which controlled for comorbid conditions. 3. QoL improved in both groups but improved significantly more in the intervention group as compared to controls. 4. The average cost of the intervention was estimated to be $216 per patient. Including the cost of intervention, costs in the control group were estimated to be $460 per patient higher, an average of $153 per patient per month over the study period. **Limitations:** 1. The 90-day follow-up period is relatively short, particularly for calculating program costs. 2. The care provided by informal caregivers was valued at only $6 per hour for the cost-benefit analysis. Patients in the intervention group required intense care by informal caregivers, and their costs may have been valued at too low a level.

Level of Focus	Reference	Setting/Population	Intervention	Results
System	Venner & Seelbinder (1996)	**Setting:** Borgess Medical Center (tertiary referral center in the Midwest) **Population:** Programwide: Physicians chose whether or not to use features of the program in the management of their patients. The number of patients enrolled is unknown.	This multidisciplinary CHF management program includes clinical pathways detailing management from admissions to post-discharge, nurse case management, and an outpatient clinic. The primary goal of case management was to prevent hospital readmission. A clinical pathway for home health care was also included. The home-health clinical pathway included education, symptom monitoring, and intravenous infusion of diuretics if needed. After hospital discharge, patients were referred to an outpatient clinic. The outpatient clinic focused on behavioral modification training, assessment of patients' social support, and improvement of physical function. Care and education in the outpatient clinic was also guided by detailed protocols. Patients were seen biweekly in the clinic for 2 months and then for a final follow-up visit. All clinic appointments included supervised exercise sessions.	1. No results were presented. **Limitations:** 1. This was a description of an intervention. No evaluation of the program was presented.

Level of Focus	Reference	Setting/Population	Intervention	Results
System	Urden (1998)	**Setting:** Butterworth Hospital (Michigan) **Population:** Memberwide, description of intervention only, no population used for evaluation. All patients hospitalized for CHF enter the clinic after discharge.	This case-management program focuses on provision of care by a multidisciplinary team in a heart failure clinic. The CHF clinic has five components: (a) inpatient consultation, education, and discharge planning; (b) outpatient monitoring; (c) outpatient infusion therapy; (d) outpatient telemanagement; and (e) linkage to community and home-care resources. A 24-hour, on-call nurse practitioner operates out of the clinic. Patients enter the clinic 1 week after hospital discharge and visit the clinic once every 3 to 6 months. Home phone calls occur twice per week for 2 to 3 weeks, every other week for a month, and monthly thereafter. Care is provided by a cardiologist, a nurse practitioner, and a nurse clinician using clinical pathways.	1. No results were presented. **Limitations:** 1. The article contains a description of the program. No evaluation results are presented. The program had been in place for less than 1 year at the time of publication.
System	Pugh et al. (1999)	**Setting:** Two hospital members of the Penn State Geisinger Health System: Hershey Medical Center (Hershey, PA) and Lehigh Valley Hospital (Allentown, PA). **Population:** Programwide, description of planned randomized trial of intervention only, no population used for evaluation. Patients ($N = 200$) will all be older than 65 years and hospitalized for CHF.	The Partners-in-Care model is a nurse case-management system for recently hospitalized CHF patients. Nurse case managers work with primary-care physicians and cardiologists collaboratively. The nurse begins with visits in the hospital and continues with outpatient visits and phone contact for 6 months after the patient's release. The program includes patient education with a specially designed workbook and discharge planning.	1. No results as presented. **Limitations:** 1. The article consists of a description of the planned intervention. No evaluation of the program was presented.

Level of Focus	Reference	Setting/Population	Intervention	Results
System	Topp et al. (1998)	**Setting:** Toledo Hospital, Toledo, Ohio **Population:** Programwide: Intervention group patients were compared to usual-care controls retrospectively ($N = 491$; 88 were in intervention group). All patients had been hospitalized for CHF.	Inpatient nurse case management was carried out based on CHF critical pathways. Nurse case manager responsibilities included ensuring continuity of care, assessing patient and family educational needs, and serving as a liaison between patients and health care providers. The case manager reviewed patients' progress daily and assured that patient care was following established critical pathways. The case manager led patient-care conferences for patients and families.	1. Average hospital length of stay was 4.6 days for case-managed patients versus 6.29 days for usual-care patients ($p < .004$). Hospital charges were \$8,512 per visit in the intervention group versus \$11,218 per visit in the control group ($p < .004$). 2. Case management had an impact on length of stay and hospitalization costs independent of the involvement of a cardiologist in the patient's care. **Limitations:** 1. The analysis did not include case-mix adjustment (patients were not randomized to treatment groups; controls were chosen retrospectively). 2. The mechanism for assignment to treatment was nonrandom and was not described in the article.

Level of Focus	Reference	Setting/Population	Intervention	Results
System	Lasater, 1996	**Setting:** Medical University of South Carolina Medical Center **Population:** Memberwide, all patients discharged from the hospital with CHF who lived in a three-county area, with 41 patients used for the evaluation.	The nurse-managed clinic was designed to follow patients after hospital discharge. The clinic involved the collaborative effort of nurses, cardiologists, dietitians, and social workers. Nurse-managed care through the clinic included cardiopulmonary assessment; weight-gain monitoring; patient education regarding medication, diet, and symptom recognition; development of an exercise program; assessment of medication compliance; assessment of the home environment; and reporting to physicians on patients' condition. Care for patients followed detailed clinical pathways.	1. After 1 year, 82% of clinic patients could name one desired effect and two negative effects of their medications. Prior to the intervention, only 40% of patients could do so. 2. Six months after implementation, hospital readmission rates dropped from 25.6% to 21.9%. Average length of stay was reduced from 7.3 days to 5.7 days. Both reductions were statistically significant. 3. Hospitalization charges were reduced by $498.48 per patient in the period following implementation of the program. **Limitations:** 1. A small sample size was used for the follow-up evaluation.
System	Paul, 1997	**Setting:** Medical University of South Carolina, Charleston **Population:** Programwide, description of intervention only; no population used for evaluation. Patients enter the clinic by referral.	A nurse-managed CHF clinic was used in caring for patients. As part of a multi-disciplinary team, the nurse practitioner maintained contact with patients by phone or in-person in the clinic and was available by phone 24 hours a day. Patients had regularly scheduled follow-up by physicians and cardiologists. Patients received education from the nurse practitioner. A pharmacist evaluated patients' medications at every visit. An educational notebook was personalized for each patient with medications and care regimens.	1. No results were presented. **Limitations:** 1. This was a description of an intervention, with no evaluation results presented.

Level of Focus	Reference	Setting/Population	Intervention	Results
System	Barrella (1998)	**Setting:** Abington Memorial Hospital (serves Medicare managed care population) **Population:** Programwide, description of intervention only. No population used for evaluation. Patients are referred to the program by case managers or physicians.	A home-care program emphasized patient and family education, assessment of social support, patient compliance, and effective medication regimens. Home-care nurses conducted initial assessments of patients and developed a care plan with patients that included instruction on when to report signs and symptoms. Care protocols were based on AHCPR guidelines for CHF management. Weekly team meetings of physicians and nurses were used to manage more complex cases. Patients had access to a 24-hour nurse line to report symptoms. The call triggered a visit from a cardiac nurse if necessary. Home administration of intravenous medications and electrocardiograph monitoring were available.	1. No results were presented. **Limitations:** 1. The article consisted of a description of the intervention only. No evaluation results were presented.

Level of Focus	Reference	Setting/Population	Intervention	Results
System	Gattis et al. (1999)	**Setting:** Cardiology clinic of Duke University Medical Center, Durham, NC **Population:** Programwide: Eligible patients were randomized into intervention or usual-care control groups ($N = 188$).	The Pharmacist in Health Failure Assessment Recommendation and Monitoring (PHARM) program involved clinical pharmacists in patient care for CHF patients. The pharmacist worked with intervention-group patients, discussing their medication regimen with them and providing patient education. The program emphasized increased ACE-inhibitor use according to clinical recommendations. Patients were provided with a phone number to contact the pharmacist with questions or in urgent situations. The pharmacist contacted patients by phone at 2, 12, and 24 weeks following the initial appointment. The pharmacist maintained contact with patients' primary-care physicians.	1. The odds of death or nonfatal heart failure event were significantly higher in the control group compared to the intervention group. Primarily this difference was due to a reduction in nonfatal heart failure events and not a decrease in mortality. 2. The intervention effect remained significant in a multivariate analysis. 3. The intervention group came closer to target doses of ACE inhibitors, but there was no significant difference between intervention and control groups in the frequency of ACE-inhibitor prescriptions. **Limitations:** 1. It is not clear how many CHF patients seen in the clinic were deemed ineligible for the intervention. 2. The follow-up period for the study was only 6 months. Sustainability of the intervention and its impact was not determined.

Level of Focus	Reference	Setting/Population	Intervention	Results
System	Rosenstein (1997)	**Setting:** Metropolitan community hospital in California, which serves Medicare managed care patients (hospital not named) **Population:** Memberwide, program implemented at the hospital level.	The program consisted of a staged CQI initiative that focused on cost-saving strategies in the treatment of CHF patients. The Clinical Resource Management (CRM) system was implemented hospital-wide to promote efficient clinical management of patients. As a part of CRM, all department chairs were provided with lists of the top 10 cost and utilization centers in their department. Department chairs were then asked to prioritize these lists and select areas for focus. CHF was chosen as the primary focus for review in the internal medicine and family practice departments. Reorganization of care for CHF patients was based on evidence-based protocols and best-practice guidelines. Standing orders for the emergency room and strategies to promote transfer of patients out of Cardiac Care Unit (CCU) beds were developed. Preprinted admission orders for CHF patients and appropriateness criteria for admission to the CCU were created. Although no formal clinical pathway for medications was designed, the program focus included emphasis on increasing ACE-inhibitor and diuretic use.	1. No evaluation results were presented. Only information regarding the process of implementation was provided. **Limitations:** 1. The article contained a description of the process of implementation only. No evaluation of the program was presented. 2. The author was a consultant hired to implement the program.

Appendix D: Literature Describing Cardiovascular Disease Management Programs in Managed Care Organizations

Hypertension

Level of Focus	Reference	Setting/Population	Intervention	Results
Patient	Cantor et al. (1985)	**Setting:** Large teaching hospital (not identified) **Population:** Programwide: A 10% sample of patients diagnosed with hypertension who had been receiving care for an average of 6 years were randomly assigned to treatment and control groups ($N = 400$).	This project was a randomized clinical trial of combinations of three educational strategies: (a) 5- to 10-minute exit interview following office visit, (b) follow-up home visit to review care instructions, and (c) a series of three small-group educational sessions.	1. Home visits represented the most expensive single intervention used. 2. The most cost-effective interventions were home visits for appointment keeping, medical regimen adherence, and blood-pressure control; exit interview for weight loss and total life-years extended; small-group meetings for hypertension life-years extended. **Limitations:** 1. The sample of 400 was divided into seven treatment arms and one control group, yielding small sample sizes.

Level of Focus	Reference	Setting/Population	Intervention	Results
Patient	Jones et al. (1987)	**Setting:** St. Luke's Hospital, Cleveland, OH **Population:** Programwide: Patients who had visited the emergency room for hypertension were randomized to control and treatment groups ($N = 72$).	This educational intervention (based on the Health Belief Model) was designed for patients who had visited the emergency room for their hypertension. Control-group patients received routine nursing care or nursing care with a follow-up phone call, whereas intervention-group patients received a Health Belief Model intervention program, or the Health Belief Model intervention program with a follow-up phone call. The Health Belief Model intervention consisted of assessment of the patient's perceived susceptibility to his or her illness, seriousness of illness, benefits of treatment, and risk of the disease process. Education was based on the results of these assessments, following the standard model framework.	1. The routine-care control group had the lowest compliance of all four groups for making and keeping follow-up appointments. 2. The Health Belief Model intervention was a statistically significant predictor of appointment making and appointment keeping. 3. The need for child care was also a statistically significant predictor of appointment making and appointment keeping. **Limitations:** 1. Small sample size: 72 patients were divided into four treatment groups, $n = 16, 17, 30,$ and 9. 2. Only patients who visited the emergency room for their hypertension were enrolled.

Level of Focus	Reference	Setting/Population	Intervention	Results
Patient	Clark et al. (1992)	**Setting:** Two large teaching hospitals (not identified) **Population:** Programwide: All eligible patients were identified through chart review; from among the eligible, all who agreed to participate were randomly assigned to treatment and control groups (N = 324).	Take Pride was a patient-education program that consisted of a 2-hour group education session for 8 to 10 adults per group held weekly for 4 weeks. The education program was based on social cognitive theory. Patients were taught problem recognition and solving through instruction, videotapes, and workbooks. Patients were taught to identify behavioral goals, develop a plan to achieve these goals, and devise a reward system for themselves. Topics covered included diet, medications, exercise, emotional well-being, rest, smoking, social relationships, communication with providers, and family interaction. Education sessions took place at the hospital.	1. After 12 months, the intervention group experienced significantly better quality of life (Hypertension, as measured by the Sickness Impact Profile) than controls. Subscales that demonstrated significant improvement in the intervention group compared to controls related to emotional behavior and alertness. 2. Women in the intervention group demonstrated significantly greater improvement in psychosocial scores, scores related to work, and alertness than women in the control group. 3. Men in the intervention group demonstrated significantly greater improvement in ambulation scores than men in the control group but no improvement in psychosocial scores. **Limitations:** 1. Volunteer bias: Of 785 eligible patients, 324 agreed to participate.

Level of Focus	Reference	Setting/Population	Intervention	Results
Provider	O'Connor et al. (1999)	**Setting:** Two primary care clinics: Clinic A, a family practice clinic in a medium-size Minnesota town with four family practice physicians; Clinic B, three separate clinics located in St. Paul, MN (part of an eight-clinic system), with three to four family-practice physicians each. **Population:** Memberwide: All patients enrolled in the clinics with a diagnosis of hypertension were affected by guideline implementation; all hypertension patients enrolled during a 12-month study period were used for evaluation ($N = 1{,}665$ for evaluation).	Hypertension care guidelines were implemented in primary-care clinics. In Clinic A, provider training was provided in hypertension guidelines, multiple checking, and standardization of blood-pressure measurement, increased awareness of documentation of blood-pressure readings by providers, development of documentation of blood-pressure measurement and patient phone-call flow sheets, improved documentation of patient medications, and a computerized patient reminder system. In Clinic B, provider training was provided in hypertension guidelines, development of implementation goals, use of a CQI team to oversee implementation of guidelines, training of nurses in blood-pressure measurement, reliance on physicians to provide patient education, a computerized patient-reminder system, and improvement in documentation of patient medication use.	1. A statistically and clinically significant improvement in the proportion of patients achieving target blood pressure 12 months after initiation of guideline implementation was observed. Statistically significant improvements were observed in both systolic and diastolic blood pressure. 2. In multivariate analysis controlling for age, gender, and number of outpatient visits, implementation of guidelines was a significant predictor of the proportion of patients with improved blood-pressure control. 3. There was no change in the proportion of patients receiving recommended hypertension medications after implementation of the guidelines. 4. The mean number of outpatient clinic visits rose significantly following implementation of the guidelines. This increase represented both physician office visits and office visits for nurse blood-pressure checks. 5. Costs were not included in this evaluation, but the increase in outpatient visits led authors to conclude that guideline implementation would lead to increased short-term costs. **Limitations:** 1. The clinics chosen for the evaluation were not representative sites. The clinics studied expressed particular interest in guideline implementation and were practice sites for physicians involved in guideline development. Success in these clinics, therefore, may not be generalizable.

Level of Focus	Reference	Setting/Population	Intervention	Results
System	Christianson et al. (1997)	**Setting:** HealthSystem Minnesota, Minneapolis, MN. **Population:** Memberwide, patients at an intervention site compared with patients at a control site.	Team management of hypertension included decentralized care by nurse coordinators, an emphasis on patient involvement in care decisions, and ongoing patient and provider education. The intervention includes continuous monitoring of patient outcomes and satisfaction.	1. No evaluation results for the intervention were reported. The article identified implementation issues encountered. **Limitations:** 1. The evaluation was limited to an assessment of implementation facilitators and obstacles.
System	Pheley et al. (1995)	**Setting:** Park Nicollet Medical Center, serving 60% HMO patients and 40% fee-for-service patients at the time of the study **Population:** Memberwide, all patients have access to the hypertension screening program. Patients can self-refer or are referred to the program by their physicians. Whereas 468 were screened for hypertension, 200 actually enrolled in program due to high blood pressure.	This evaluation focuses on a nurse-managed hypertension screening and management program that has been in place since 1972. Patients who present to the clinic and are already taking hypertension medications, or who have elevated blood pressure, are entered into the management program. The program includes patient education about diet, alcohol, and exercise. All screening results are forwarded to the primary-care physician, who makes all treatment decisions. Blood-pressure measurements are taken from all patients every 2 to 3 weeks until normotensive status is reached. During this time, patients also receive one-on-one counseling with the nurse. An automated database generates mailed reminders to patients to encourage compliance with care regimens and appointment keeping.	1. A significant improvement in the number of individuals with blood pressure in control after 12 months was demonstrated among both patients using and not using hypertension medications. 2. There was a significant decrease in both systolic and diastolic blood-pressure measures for individuals using and not using medication after 12 months. **Limitations:** 1. The population was predominantly white and middle class. 2. A high dropout rate in the management program was noted: 48.9% of those enrolled in the program dropped out. Final outcomes are based on a sample of only 108 patients.

229

Level of Focus	Reference	Setting/Population	Intervention	Results
System	Schultz et al. (1994)	**Setting:** Hypertension Clinic at the Mayo Memorial Clinic, Rochester, MN **Population:** Memberwide, no population used for evaluation.	A nurse-managed clinic that offered multidisciplinary team care for hypertension. The clinic offered care to three types of patients: (a) short-term patients, (b) patients receiving liver transplants, and (c) long-term patients. Intervention was tailored for each type of patient and included some combination of the following nurse-provided services: blood-pressure monitoring three times daily for inpatients, patient education and dietary counseling, coordination of outpatient appointments, test-result review and follow-up, immunosuppression education (for transplant patients), monitoring of side effects, and database monitoring of patient data. All three groups of patients received a dietitian consult and were taught home blood-pressure monitoring and provided with all necessary equipment.	1. No evaluation of the intervention was reported. **Limitations:** 1. The article contained only a description of the intervention.

Level of Focus	Reference	Setting/Population	Intervention	Results
System	Gerber & Stewart (1998)	**Setting:** West Baltimore, MD **Population:** Community-wide.	The Baltimore Alliance for the Prevention and Control of Hypertension and Diabetes was a community-based program that includes the joint efforts of the University of Maryland School of Medicine Center for Health Policy Research, the Joslin Diabetes Center, several MCO partners, Legacy 2000 (a Baltimore newspaper's male health initiative), Millennium Healthcare (a health education and services organization), and a pharmaceutical company (Hoechst Marion Roussel). The program involved the use of community health workers and was modeled on the Barefoot Doctor program in China. Church-based education and screening were used to enroll patients in treatment programs. The program was designed to mobilize the community in the management of hypertension and diabetes and to provide culturally relevant care. Care included stepped, achievable goals that encouraged patients to take control of their own disease management.	1. No assessment of the intervention was reported. **Limitations:** 1. The article is a description of the intervention only.

231

Anticoagulants

Level of Focus	Reference	Setting/Population	Intervention	Results
System	Seabrook et al. (1990)	**Setting:** Academic hospital (not identified) **Population:** Memberwide: All patients hospitalized requiring long-term anticoagulant therapy were entered into the clinic ($N = 93$).	The intervention was a hospital-based, nurse-managed anticoagulation clinic. Patients received educational information from nurse clinicians prior to discharge, including education regarding signs of complications. No restrictions were placed on diet, activity, or lifestyle. Patients received prothrombin measurements one to three times per week until a therapeutic dosage was achieved. Nurse follow-up continued through phone contact. Noncompliant patients were referred to their primary-care physicians for further follow-up.	1. Patients received the intervention for an average of 40 months, with an average of five medication-dosage changes per patient. 2. No anticoagulant-related deaths or venous thrombotic events occurred during the study period. The complication rate was 3.2 per 1,000 patient-months of the treatment for hemorrhagic complications and 5.3 per 1,000 patient-months for major bleeding events. **Limitations:** 1. It is difficult to evaluate program success without an external comparison group or comparison to a previous time period.
System	Becker et al. (1994)	**Setting:** University of Virginia Health Sciences Center, Charlottesville, VA, and the University of California at Davis Medical Center **Population:** Unknown if program- or memberwide. The University of Virginia clinic cares for 250 patients; the UC Davis clinic cares for 300 patients.	Nurse practitioner-managed anticoagulation clinics used portable prothrombin-time monitors for patients. Nurses tested times, conducted patient evaluation and made adjustments in warfarin therapy. Nurse practitioners at both sites maintained computerized patient databases, arranged follow-up appointments, and contacted patients by phone for follow-up. Nurse practitioners also arranged home care for patients, if necessary.	1. Clinics at both sites achieved prothrombin times near the therapeutic range. 2. Complication rates did not differ at the two sites. Rates were 1.0%, 1.5%, and 5.9% for fatal bleeding, life-threatening bleeding, and recurrent thromboembolism. **Limitations:** 1. The authors do not describe how the patient population was referred to the clinic. Therefore, it cannot be determined if the clinics were member- or programwide. 2. Outcomes assessment was not placed in any comparative context, so it is difficult to determine if this intervention should be considered successful.

Level of Focus	Reference	Setting/Population	Intervention	Results
System	Bussey et al. (1989)	**Setting:** Brady-Green Community Health Center, San Antonio, TX **Population:** Programwide: Patients are referred to clinic from the medical center's hospital or from any affiliated outpatient clinics (N = 231 seen in clinic; n = 89 used in evaluation).	The intervention consisted of a pharmacist-managed anticoagulation clinic. Patients were provided with an information booklet, a dosing calendar, and emergency phone-contact numbers at their first visit. Patients were educated about signs of complications and the importance of compliance with medications. Patients were initially seen at 1- and 2-week intervals. Once stabilized, patients were seen at 4- to 6-week intervals. Frequency of visits was determined by the pharmacist.	1. During the follow-up (all patients were followed for 1 to 2 years), 4 patients experienced major hemorrhagic events, 20 experienced minor hemorrhagic events, and 5 experienced thromboembolic events. 2. Duration of therapy was not related to occurrence of adverse events. **Limitations:** 1. Patients were referred to the clinic from hospital and outpatient settings. It is difficult to determine the population denominator. 2. Of 231 patients seen in the clinic over the evaluation time period, 149 were excluded from the study because they had less than 7 months of continuous monitoring. 3. There was no control group.

Level of Focus	Reference	Setting/Population	Intervention	Results
System	Wilt et al. (1995)	**Setting:** Family Practice Medical Group, Inc., in Gainesville, FL, affiliated with the University of Florida. **Population:** Programwide: Patients followed by the Anticoagulation Monitoring Service (AMS) were compared to nonrandom control patients followed only by family-practice physicians ($N = 112$).	AMS was a pharmacist-managed anticoagulation clinic for patients on warfarin. New patients were seen weekly and then biweekly until they were stabilized. All stable patients were seen at 4- to 6-week intervals. Patients were provided with written and verbal education about warfarin and were questioned extensively at each visit about complications and side effects. PT and INRs were measured at regular intervals. Patients who missed appointments in the clinic were called to reschedule.	1. There were significantly more major hemorrhagic events in the control group as compared to the AMS group, but this occurred only among patients with major comorbidities and noncompliant patients in each group. 2. The control group also had significantly more unplanned clinic visits, emergency-room visits, and hospital admissions than the AMS group. 3. A cost savings of $4,072.68 per person-year of follow-up reportedly would have been achieved if the control-group patients were seen in the AMS. **Limitations:** 1. Extensive comparison of the control and AMS groups at baseline was not provided. 2. Patients were retrospectively identified as having been in the control or treatment group. It is not clear what factors led patients to be treated in the AMS or by family-practice providers.

Level of Focus	Reference	Setting/Population	Intervention	Results
System	Conte et al. (1986)	**Setting:** San Francisco General Hospital Medical Center **Population:** Programwide: Patients treated in the San Francisco General Hospital Medical Center were referred to the clinic by their physicians or after inpatient treatment (N = 141).	A pharmacist-managed anticoagulation clinic was established in 1974. The clinic operated 2 half days per week. Patients were referred to the clinic from general or specialty clinics or at hospital discharge. Patients met with a pharmacist, but a cardiologist was available for consultation. Pharmacists interviewed patients for information about diet, prescriptions, and comorbidities and provided extensive education about warfarin treatment. The pharmacist also performed a physical exam. Prothrombin (PT) and other laboratory tests were ordered by the pharmacists. Patients continued to be followed by their own physicians, and the clinic pharmacist maintained communication with primary-care physicians.	1. Over the 9-year evaluation period, 60% of PTs were within therapeutic range. 2. Only four major hemorrhagic events occurred during the evaluation period (.002 events per patient-month). 3. Eighty-nine minor hemorrhagic events (.05 per patient-month) occurred during the evaluation period. 4. About 37% of patients were determined to be noncompliant. **Limitations:** 1. The population served is unclear. Patients treated within the medical center were referred to the clinic at physicians' discretion. It is not clear what portion of patients who seek care at the medical center for anticoagulation were referred to and enrolled in the clinic. 2. This article reviewed clinic results between 1974 and 1984 approximately. This predates the widespread proliferation of managed care and may have primarily occurred in a fee-for-service environment.

Other Cardiovascular Disease (CVD)

Level of Focus	Reference	Setting/Population	Intervention	Results
System	DeBusk et al. (1994)	**Setting:** Five Kaiser Permanente Medical Centers in the San Francisco Bay Area **Population:** Programwide, intervention group patients compared to randomized control group (N = 585).	A case-management program for patients hospitalized with acute myocardial infarction was implemented in the five medical centers. Initial patient education by a nurse case manager for smoking cessation, diet, and exercise began during the inpatient stay. Patients received physician-provided smoking-cessation counseling, a relapse-prevention manual, and a relaxation tape. The nurse case manager scheduled regular smoking-cessation support phone calls for 6 months following discharge. Patients received education about diet and were placed on lipid-lowering drugs if necessary. Patients received exercise training and were telephoned for exercise monitoring regularly for 6 months.	1. Biochemically verified smoking-cessation rates were significantly higher in the intervention group at 6 and 12 months after intervention. 2. Both intervention and control groups demonstrated reduced consumption of cholesterol and saturated fat. 3. Significantly more intervention-group patients were on lipid-lowering therapy at 6 and 12 months following the intervention. 4. LDL and total cholesterol values decreased to a significantly greater degree among intervention-group patients. **Limitations:** 1. The control group also received smoking-cessation and dietary counseling as inpatients. A smoking-cessation program was offered to control-group patients at a cost of $50. About 5% of control-group patients also participated in an exercise program at significant cost. 2. The 1-year follow-up period did not include mortality or reoccurrence of myocardial infarction as outcome measures.

Level of Focus	Reference	Setting/Population	Intervention	Results
System	Anderson et al. (1997)	**Setting:** St. Luke's Episcopal Hospital and the affiliated Texas Heart Institute, Houston, TX **Population:** Memberwide.	A CQI initiative was undertaken due to the growing pressures of managed care and the desire to maintain dominance in the area of CVD management. The initiative involved development of a Service Line Management staff assigned to the coordination and oversight of care provided to all CVD patients. The Service Line Management staff were responsible for (a) clinical management, (b) business management, and (c) promotion. Several committees were developed, each headed by a physician and a member of the Service Line Management staff. These committees were intended to advise the Service Line Management Committee, which met regularly to coordinate the work of these committees. The initiative included development and implementation of practice guidelines, establishment of quality indicators, review of adherence to guidelines, and review of patient outcomes. Outcomes management for CVD focused primarily on eliminating variations in practice patterns. The hospital established global package-pricing programs and partnerships with payers and providers for the care of CVD patients.	1. The hospital received a 90% rating on patient QoL using the Press Ganey system. 2. Risk-adjusted mortality and morbidity rates at the hospital were within population norms. 3. The hospital was successful in altering physician practice patterns, resulting in more timely transfer of patients out of Intensive Care Unit beds. **Limitations:** 1. The evaluation was informal in nature. 2. No evidence of any impact on patient health outcomes was reported.

Dyslipidemia

Level of Focus	Reference	Setting/Population	Intervention	Results
System	Chima et al. (1990)	**Setting:** Cleveland Clinic Foundation, Cleveland, OH **Population:** Programwide: Patients seeking care at the Cleveland Clinic Foundation could choose lipid management through the Lipid Management Clinic if they desired intensive treatment ($N = 291$).	The Lipid Management Clinic focused on application of National Cholesterol Education Project (NCEP) guidelines. This article describes, in particular, the nutritional intervention provided by the clinic. Patients saw a nutritionist in the clinic at baseline, 6 weeks, and 12 weeks. Prior to each visit, dietary diaries were analyzed by a computer program. Patients received individual counseling for diet modification and a stepped approach to dietary change was emphasized.	1. The greatest change in diet occurred after the initial visit and was maintained to the 12-week visit. 2. Patients reduced their intake of cholesterol, calories from fat, and calories from saturated fat. 3. LDL cholesterol levels were significantly reduced after 3 months. There were no statistically significant changes in HDL or triglyceride levels. Limitations: 1. This study focused only on the nutritional counseling component of the clinic. 2. Volunteer bias: Patients were not routinely referred to the clinic but opted to attend if they desired intensive treatment. The population was described by the authors as highly motivated to change their dietary habits. 3. There was no formal evaluation of the program but rather a brief summary of data. 4. It is not clear if patients' dietary modifications were maintained after their final clinic visit (12 weeks after baseline).

Level of Focus	Reference	Setting/Population	Intervention	Results
System	La Forge et al. (1996)	**Setting:** San Diego Cardiac Center Medical Group **Population:** Programwide: Patients were referred from within the cardiac center and also from external sources. The center contracted with several HMOs. At the time of publication, 350 patients were enrolled, but this is a description of the program only; no population was used for evaluation.	The nurse-managed lipid-management program provided care using a multidisciplinary team approach. The care team included a clinic coordinator, cardiologists, nurses, a dietitian, and an exercise specialist. Program elements were based on NCEP guidelines for care. All new clinic patients received a health and lifestyle assessment by a physician. Patients received dietary and weight-loss counseling from the nutritionist, exercise counseling, and stress-management counseling. Exercise programs are held on-site for patients. Pharmacological management, including management of patient compliance with medications, was a central feature of the program. Coordination of all clinic services by a nurse clinic manager was also considered a key to the success of the program.	1. No evaluation results were provided. **Limitations:** 1. Patients were referred to the clinic from internal and external physicians. It is not clear what the population denominator was. 2. Description of the intervention only. No formal evaluation results were presented.

Appendix E: Literature Describing Arthritis Management Programs in Managed Care Organizations

Level of Focus	Reference	Setting/Population	Intervention	Results
Patient	Fries et al. (1997)	**Setting:** Patients from three settings: Group Health (Seattle), three Northern California rheumatology clinics, and patients participating in Healthtrac, a general health-education program, who self-identified as having arthritis **Population:** Programwide, intervention groups from three sites compared to control groups from the same sites ($N = 809$).	This intervention is a by-mail arthritis self-management program for patients with osteoarthritis and rheumatoid arthritis. By-mail health-assessment questionnaires completed by each patient were used to create computer-generated letters signed by the patient's physician, which detail the patient's condition, progress, and physician recommendations for care. Recommendations were tailored to each patient based on age, level of disability, education, medication regimen, pain, and self-efficacy. Patients were also mailed the *Arthritis Help Book*, a relaxation audio tape, an exercise video, and information regarding medication side effects. Patient progress reports and physician letters were generated at 3-month intervals for 6 months.	1. Intervention-group patients showed positive, significant improvement, both compared to baseline and compared to controls, in function, global vitality, tender-joint count, exercise frequency, and personal self-efficacy (confidence) 6 months after the intervention. Both intervention-group participants and controls demonstrated significant improvements in pain. 2. Intervention-group participants reported significantly fewer sick days/days at home 6 months after the intervention as compared to baseline. 3. Intervention-group patients had significantly fewer doctor visits, both compared to baseline and compared to controls, in the 6 months following the intervention. 4. These findings were generally consistent across all three patient cohorts. 5. At 1 year, the intervention-group members continued to improve in painful-joint count and exercise frequency. Controls, who were entered into the program at 6 months, demonstrated the same improvements that the original intervention group displayed at 6 months. **Limitations:** 1. The follow-up period was only 6 months. 2. Patients were asked to recall the number of their doctor visits and number of sick days over a 6-month period. 3. The statistical analysis was limited to paired sample t tests.

Level of Focus	Reference	Setting/Population	Intervention	Results
System	Schned et al. (1995)	**Setting:** Rheumatology Treatment and Resource Center of Park Nicollet Clinic, Minneapolis, Minnesota **Population:** Programwide, eligible patients randomized to treatment and control groups (N = 107).	The intervention consisted of a multidisciplinary care team for patients with early-stage rheumatoid arthritis (patients with advanced rheumatoid arthritis, osteoarthritis, or lupus are not included in the program). Primary care for the patient was provided by a rheumatologist who worked in conjunction with a care team. The care team included a rheumatologist, mental health specialist, social worker, podiatrist, head outpatient nurse, dietician, physical therapist, and occupational therapist, all of whom provided care to the patient on the primary provider's referral. The care team met monthly to review all new patients in the program and quarterly to review all enrolled patients. Patients and their families and friends participated in a half-day education and management program, and patients engaged in a detailed phone-assessment interview at enrollment to identify patient-specific problems. This interview was repeated every 3 months. A formal written Arthritis Care Plan was developed for each patient and continuously updated by providers.	1. After 1 year, no difference between treatment and control groups in painful-joint count, duration of morning stiffness, ACR functional class, fatigue, or presence of nodules was observed. 2. After 1 year, no difference between groups in physical functioning (as measured by the HAQ), satisfaction with physical functioning, mobility, physical activity, dexterity, or pain were observed. 3. After 1 year, no differences between groups in depression, perception of helplessness, life satisfaction, or global arthritis rating were observed. 4. After 1 year, no significant differences between groups in use of medications, number of outpatient visits, number of tests ordered, hospitalizations, surgical procedures, use of nontraditional treatment, or use of aids/devices were observed. **Limitations:** 1. The population was primarily white, well-educated, affluent, and insured. 2. The same team members treated both intervention- and control-group patients. There may have been some spillover effect of the intervention onto the control-group patients.

References

Abourizk, N. N., O'Connor, P. J., Crabtree, B. F., & Schnatz, J. D. (1994). An outpatient model of integrated diabetes treatment and education: Functional, metabolic, and knowledge outcomes. *The Diabetes Educator, 20*(5), 416-421.

Abraham, W. T., & Bristow, M. R. (1997). Specialized centers for heart failure management [Editorial]. *Circulation, 96*(9), 2755-2757.

Agency for Health Care Policy and Research (AHCPR). (1994). Heart failure: Management of patients with left-ventricular systolic dysfunction. *Clinical Practice Guidlines: Quick Reference Guide for Clinicians,* No. 11, 1-25.

Anderson, J., Nangle, M., & Alexander, W. A. (1997). Cardiovascular outcomes management and managed care contracting: Experience from St. Luke's Episcopal Hospital and the Texas Heart Institute. *Critical Care Nursing Quarterly, 19*(4), 48-55.

Anderson, R. M. (1995). Patient empowerment and the traditional medical model: A case of irreconcilable differences? *Diabetes Care, 18*(3), 412-415.

Anderson, R. M., Funnell, M. M., Butler, P. M., Arnold, M. S., Fitzgerald, J. T., & Feste, C. C. (1995). Patient empowerment: Results of a randomized controlled trial. *Diabetes Care, 18*(7), 943-949.

Arnold, S. B., Byrd, R. C., Meister, W., Melmon, K., Cheitlin, M. D., Bristow, J. D., Parmley, W. W., & Chatterjee, K. (1980). Long-term digitalis therapy improves left ventricular function in heart failure. *New England Journal of Medicine, 303*(25), 1443-1448.

Aubert, R. E., Herman, W. H., Waters, J., Moore, W., Sutton, D., Peterson, B. L., Bailey, C. M., & Koplan, J. P. (1998). Nurse case management to improve glycemic control in diabetic patients in a health maintenance organization: A randomized, controlled trial. *Annals of Internal Medicine, 129*(8), 605-612.

Aucott, J. N., Pelecanos, E., Dombrowski, R., Fuehrer, S. M., Laich, J., & Aron, D. C. (1996). Implementation of local guidelines for cost-effective management of hypertension; A trial of the firm system. *Journal of General Internal Medicine, 11*(3), 139-146.

Australia/New Zealand Heart Failure Research Collaborative Group. (1997). Randomised placebo-controlled trial of carvedilol in patients with congestive heart failure due to ischaemic heart disease. *Lancet, 349,* 375-380.

Barlow, J. H., & Barefoot, J. (1996). Group education for people with arthritis. *Patient Education and Counseling, 27*(3), 257-267.

Barrella, P., & Monica, E. D. (1998). Managing congestive heart failure at home. *AACN Clinical Issues, 9*(3), 377-388.

Basler, H. D. (1993). Group treatment for pain and discomfort. *Patient Education and Counseling, 20*(2-3), 167-175.

Beary, J. F., Benson, H., & Klemchuk, H. (1974). A simple psychophysiologic technique which elicits the hypometabolic changes of the relaxation response. *Psychosomatic Medicine, 36,* 115-120.

Becker, A., McGhan, S., Dolovich, J., Proudlock, M., & Mitchell, I. (1994). Essential ingredients for an ideal education program for children with asthma and their families. *Chest, 106* (4 Suppl), 231S-234S.

Becker, D. M., DeMong, L. K., Kaplan, P., Hutchinson, R., Callahan, C. M., Fihn, S. D., & White, R. H. (1994). Anticoagulation therapy and primary care internal medicine: A nurse practitioner model for combined clinical science. *Journal of General Internal Medicine, 9*(9), 525-527.

Belardinelli, R., Georgiou, D., Scocco, V., Barstow, T. J., & Purcaro, A. (1995). Low intensity exercise training in patients with chronic heart failure. *Journal of the American College of Cardiology, 26*(4), 975-982.

Benjamin, E. M., Schneider, M. S., & Hinchey, K. T. (1999). Implementing practice guidelines for diabetes care using problem-based learning: A prospective controlled trial using firm systems. *Diabetes Care, 22*(10), 1672-1678.

Berg, C. E., Alt, K. J., Himmel, J. K., & Judd, B. J. (1985). The effects of patient education on patient cognition and dis-related anxiety. *Patient Education and Counseling, 7*(4), 389-394.

Bill-Harvey, D., Rippey, R., Abeles, M., Donald, M. J., Downing, D., Ingenito, F., & Pfeiffer, C. A. (1989). Outcome of an osteoarthritis education program for low-literacy patients taught by indigenous instructors. *Patient Education and Counseling, 13*(2), 133-142.

Bilodeau, A. (1995). Easing the pain of arthritis. *HMO, 36*(4), 70-74.

Boggs, P. B., Hayati, F., Washburne, W. F., & Wheeler, D. A. (1999). Using statistical process control charts for the continual improvement of asthma care. *The Joint Commission Journal on Quality Improvement, 25*(4), 163-181.

Brass-Mynderse, N. J. (1996). Disease management for chronic congestive heart failure. *The Journal of Cardiovascular Nursing, 11*(1), 54-62.

Brosnan, J. (1996). A patient-focused pathway for ambulatory anticoagulation care. *Journal of Nursing Care Quality, 11*(2). 41-53.

Buchner, D. A., Butt, L. T. De Stefano, A., Edgren, B., Suarez, A., & Evans, R. M. (1998). Effects of an asthma management program on the asthmatic member: Patient-centered results of a 2-year study in a managed care organization. *American Journal of Managed Care, 4*(9), 1288-1297.

Bussey, H. I., Rospond, R. M., Quandt, C. M., & Clark, G. M. (1989). The safety and effectiveness of long-term warfarin therapy in an anticoagulation clinic. *Pharmacotherapy, 9*(4), 214-219.

Calfas, K. J., Kaplan, R. M., & Ingram, R. E. (1992). One-year evaluation of cognitive-behavioral intervention in osteoarthritis. *Arthritis Care and Research 5*(4), 202-209.

Cantor, J. C., Morisky, D. E., Green, L. W., Levine, D. M., & Salkever, D. S. (1985). Cost-effectiveness of educational interventions to improve patient outcomes in blood pressure control. *Preventive Medicine, 14*(6), 782-800.

Chicoye, L., Roethel, C. R., Hatch, M. H., & Wesolowski, W. (1998). Diabetes care management: A managed care approach. *WMJ, 97*(3), 32-34.

Chima, C. S., Miller-Kovach, K., Zeller, M., Cook, K., & Schupp, K. (1990). Lipid management clinic: Dietary intervention for patients with hypercholesterolemia. *Journal of the American Dietetic Association, 90*(2), 272-274.

Chiquette, E., Amato, M. G., & Bussey, H. I. (1998). Comparison of an anticoagulation clinic with usual medical care: Anticoagulation control, patient outcomes, and health care costs. *Archives of Internal Medicine, 158*(15), 1641-1647.

Christianson, J. B., Pietz, L., Taylor, R., Woolley, A., & Knutson, D. J. (1997). Implementing programs for chronic illness management: The case of hypertension services. *The Joint Commission Journal on Quality Improvement, 23*(11), 593-601.

Cintron, G., Bigas, C., Linares, E., Aranda, J. M., & Hernandez, E. (1983). Nurse practitioner role in a chronic congestive heart failure clinic: In-hospital time, costs, and patient satisfaction. *Heart Lung, 12*(3), 237-240.

Clark, N. M., Feldman, C. H., Evans, D., Millman, E. J., Wailewski, Y., & Valle, I. (1981). The effectiveness of education for family management of asthma in children: A preliminary report. *Health Education Quarterly, 8*(2), 166-174.

Clark, N. M., Janz, N. K., Becker, M. H., Schork, M. A., Wheeler, J., Liang, J., Dodge, J. A., Keteyian, S., Rhoads, K. L., & Santinga, J. T. (1992). Impact of self-management education on the functional health status of older adults with heart disease. *Gerontologist, 32*(4), 438-443.

Coats, A. J., Adamopoulos, S., Radaelli, A., McCance, A., Meyer, T. E., Bernardi, L., Solda, P. L., Davey, P., Ormerod, O., & Forfar, C. (1992). Controlled trial of physical training in chronic heart failure: Exercise performance, hemodynamics, ventilation, and autonomic function. *Circulation, 85*(6), 2119-2131.

Cofer, L. A. (1997). Aggressive cholesterol management: Role of the lipid nurse specialist. *Heart Lung, 26*(5), 337-344.

Cohen, J. L., Sauter, S. V., DeVellis, R. F., & DeVellis, B. M. (1986). Evaluation of arthritis self-management courses led by laypersons and by professionals. *Arthritis and Rheumatism, 29*(3), 388-393.

Cohn, J. N. (1996). The management of chronic heart failure. *New England Journal of Medicine, 335*(7), 490-498.

Cohn, J. N., Archibald, D. G., Ziesche, S., Franciosa, J. A., Harston, W. E., Tristani, F. E., Dunkman, W. B., Jacobs, W., Francis, G. S., & Flohr, K. H. (1986). Effect of vasodilator therapy on mortality in chronic congestive heart failure: Results of a Veterans Administration Cooperative Study. *New England Journal of Medicine, 314*(24), 1547-1552.

Cohn, J. N., Johnson, G., Ziesche, S., Cobb, F., Francis, G., Tristani, F., Smith, R., Dunkman, W. B., Loeb, H., & Wong, M. (1991). A comparison of enalapril with hydralazine-isosorbide dinitrate in the treatment of chronic congestive heart failure. *New England Journal of Medicine, 325*(5), 303-310. (see comments)

CONSENSUS Trial Study Group. (1987). Effects of Enalapril on mortality in severe congestive heart failure: Results of the Cooperative North Scandinavian Enalaril Survival Study (CONSENSUS). *New England Journal of Medicine, 316,* 1429-1435.

Conte, R. R., Kehoe, W. A., Nielson, N., & Lodhia, H. (1986). Nine-year experience with a pharmacist-managed anticoagulation clinic. *American Journal of Hospital Pharmacy, 43*(10), 2460-2464.

Creer, T. L., Backial, M., Burns, K. L., Leung, P., Marion, R. J., Miklich, D. R., Morrill, C., Taplin, P. S., & Ullman, S. (1988). Living with asthma: I. Genesis and development of a self-management program for childhood asthma. *The Journal of Asthma, 25*(6), 335-362.

Davidson, M. B. (1997). Diabetes management: Improving care in HMO and community settings. *Medical Interface, 10*(8), 86-90.

Davis, P., Busch, A. J., Lowe, J. C., Taniguchi, J., & Djkowich, B. (1994). Evaluation of a rheumatoid arthritis patient education program: Impact on knowledge and self-efficacy. *Patient Education and Counseling, 24*(1), 55-61. (see comments)

DeBusk, R. F., Miller, N. H., Superko, H. R., Dennis, C. A., Thomas, R. J., Lew, H. T., Berger, W. E., Heller, R. S., Rompf, J., & Gee, D. (1994). A case-management system for coronary risk factor modification after acute myocardial infarction. *Annals of Internal Medicine, 120*(9), 721-729. (see comments)

The Diabetes Control and Complications Trial Research Group. (1993). The effect of intensive treatment of diabetes on the development and progression of long-term complications in insulin-dependent diabetes mellitus. *New England Journal of Medicine, 329*(14), 977-986.

Domurat, E. S. (1999). Diabetes managed care and clinical outcomes: The Harbor City, California, Kaiser Permanente Diabetes Care System. *American Journal of Managed Care, 5,* 1299-1307.

Dracup, K. Baker, D. W., Dunbar, S. B., Dacey, R. A., Brooks, N. H., Johnson, J. C., Oken, C., & Massie, B. M. (1994). Management of heart failure: II. Counseling, education, and lifestyle modifications. *Journal of the American Medical Association, 272,* 1442-1446.

Edelstein, E. L., & Cesta, T. G. (1993). Nursing case management: An innovative model of care for hospitalized patients with diabetes. *The Diabetes Educator, 19*(6), 517-521.

Ellenbecker, C. H., Garcia, I., & Kane, M. (1998). State contracting initiatives for quality improvement in asthma care. *Journal for Healthcare Quality, 20*(4), 4-10.

Etzwiler, D. D. (1972). The patient is a member of the medical team. *Journal of the American Dietetic Association, 61*(4), 421-423.

Fitzgerald, J. F., Smith, D. M., Martin, D. K., Freedman, J. A., & Katz, B. P. (1994). A case manager intervention to reduce readmissions. *Archives of Internal Medicine, 154*(15), 1721-1729.

Follath, F., Cleland, J. G., Klein, W., & Murphy, R. (1998). Etiology and response to drug treatment in heart failure. *Journal of the American College of Cardiology, 32*(5), 1167-1172.

Forshee, J. D., Whalen, E. B., Hackel, R., Butt, L. T., Smeltzer, P. A., Martin, J., Lavin, P. T., & Buchner, D. A. (1998). The effectiveness of one-on-one nurse education on the outcomes of high-risk adult and pediatric patients with asthma. *Managed Care Interface, 11*(12), 82-92.

Franz, M. J., Monk, A., Barry, B., McClain, K., Weaver, T., Cooper, N., Upham, P., Bergenstal, R., & Mazze, R. S. (1995). Effectiveness of medical nutrition therapy provided by dietitians in the management of non-insulin-dependent diabetes mellitus: A randomized, controlled clinical trial. *Journal of the American Dietetic Association, 95*(9), 1009-1017.

Friedman, N. (1996). Diabetes and managed care: The Lovelace health system's Episodes of Care program. *Managed Care Quarterly, 4*(1), 43-49.

Friedman, N. M., Gleeson, J. M., Kent, M. J., Foris, M., & Rodriguez, D. J. (1998). Management of diabetes mellitus in the Lovelace health systems' Episodes of Care program. *Effective Clinical Practice, 1*(1), 5-11.

Fries, J. F., Carey, C., & McShane, D. J. (1997). Patient education in arthritis: Randomized controlled trial of a mail-delivered program. *The Journal of Rheumatology, 24*(7), 1378-1383.

Funke Kupper, A. J., Fintelman, H., Huige, M. C., Koolen, J. J., Liem, K. L., & Lustermans, F. A. (1986). Cross-over comparison of the fixed combination of hydrochlorothiazide and triamterene and the free combination of furosemide and triamterene in the maintenance treatment of congestive heart failure. *European Journal of Clinical Pharmacology, 30*(3), 341-343.

Garabedian-Ruffalo, S. M., Gray, D. R., Sax, M. J., & Ruffalo R. L. (1985). Retrospective evaluation of a pharmacist-managed warfarin anticoagulation clinic. *American Journal of Hospital Pharmacy, 42*(2), 304-308.

Gattis, W. A., Hasselblad, V., Whellan, D. J., & O'Connor, C. M. (1999). Reduction in heart failure events by the addition of a clinical pharmacist to the heart failure management team: Results of the Pharmacist in Heart Failure Assessment Recommendation and Monitoring (PHARM) study. *Archives of Internal Medicine, 159*(16), 1939-1945.

Geffner, D. L. (1992). Diabetes care in health maintenance organizations. *Diabetes Care, 15*(Suppl 1), 44-50.

Gerber, J. (1997). Implementing quality assurance programs in multigroup practices for treating hypercholesterolemia in patients with coronary artery disease. *The American Journal of Cardiology, 80*(8B), 57H-61H.

Gerber, J. C., & Stewart, D. L. (1998). Prevention and control of hypertension and diabetes in an underserved population through community outreach and disease management: A plan of action. *Journal of the Association for Academic Minority Physicians, 9*(3), 48-52.

Gerber, R. A., Liu, G., & McCombs, J. S. (1998). Impact of pharmacist consultations provided to patients with diabetes on healthcare costs in a health maintenance organization. *American Journal of Managed Care, 4*(7), 991-1000.

Gilmet, G. P., Mallon, R. P., Griffin, B. T., & Lewandowski, J. J. (1998). The use of an integrated clinical laboratory and pharmacy diabetes database to provide physician performance feedback in an IPA-model HMO. *The Journal of Ambulatory Care Management, 21*(1), 12-23.

Ginsberg, B. H., Tan, M. H., Mazze, R., & Bergelson, A. (1998). Staged diabetes management: Computerizing a disease state management program. *Journal of Medical Systems, 22*(2), 77-87.

Goeppinger, J., Arthur, M. W., Baglioni, A. J., Jr., Brunk, S. E., & Brunner, C. M. (1989). A reexamination of the effectiveness of self-care education for persons with arthritis. *Arthritis and Rheumatism, 32*(6), 706-716.

Goeppinger, J., & Lorig, K. (1997). Interventions to reduce the impact of chronic disease: Community-based arthritis patient education. *Annual Review of Nursing Research, 15*, 101-122.

Goonan, K. J., Healy, J. M., Jr., Jordan, H. S., Zazzali, J. L., & Horowitz, M. (1993). Strategic planning applied to quality in asthma management for children. *Managed Care Quarterly, 1*(2), 62-75.

Graff, W. L., Bensussen-Walls, W., Cody, E., & Williamson, J. (1995). Population management in an HMO: New roles for nursing [see comments]. *Public Health Nursing, 12*(4), 213-221.

Greineder, D. K., Loane, K. C., & Parks, P. (1995). Reduction in resource utilization by an asthma outreach program. *Archives of Pediatric & Adolescent Medicine, 149*(4), 415-420.

Greineder, D. K., Loane, K. C., & Parks, P. (1999). A randomized controlled trial of a pediatric asthma outreach program. *The Journal of Allergy and Clinical Immunology, 103*(3 Part 1), 436-440.

Griffin, K. W., McNabb, W. L., & Shields, M. C. (1989). Telephone instruction as an adjunct to patient education of children with asthma. *Journal of Healthcare Education and Training, 4*(1), 1-6.

Hawley, D. J. (1995). Psycho-educational interventions in the treatment of arthritis. *Baillieres Clinical Rheumatology, 9*(4), 803-823.

Heinen, L., Peterson, E., Pion, K., & Leatherman, S. (1993). Quality evaluation in a managed care system: Comparative data to assess health plan performance. *Managed Care Quarterly, 1*(1), 62-76.

Hendricson, W. D., Wood, P. R., Hidalgo, H. A., Kromer, M. E., Parcel, G. S., & Ramirez, A. G. (1994). Implementation of a physician education intervention: The Childhood Asthma Project. *Archives of Pediatric & Adolescent Medicine, 148*(6), 595-601.

Hendricson, W. D., Wood, P. R., Hidalgo, H. A., Ramirez, A. G., Kromer, M. E., Selva, M., & Parcel, G. (1996). Implementation of individualized patient education for Hispanic children with asthma. *Patient Education and Counseling, 29*(2), 155-165.

Hindi-Alexander, M. C. & Cropp, G. J. (1984). Evaluation of a family asthma program. *The Journal of Allergy and Clinical Immunology, 74*(4, Part 1), 505-510.
Hirano, P. C., Laurent, D. D., & Lorig, K. (1994). Arthritis patient education studies, 1987-1991): A review of the literature. *Patient Education and Counseling, 24*(1), 9-54.
Homer, C. J. (1997). Asthma disease management (Editorial, comment). *New England Journal of Medicine, 337*(20), 1461-1463.
Institute for Clinical Systems Improvement (ICSI). (1998). *ICSI health care guideline: Congestive heart failure in adults.* Minneapolis, MN: Author.
Jacobs, R. P. (1998). Hypertension and managed care. *American Journal of Managed Care, 4*(12 Suppl), S749-S752.
Jones, P. K., Jones, S. L., & Katz, J. (1987a). Improving compliance for asthmatic patients visiting the emergency department using a health belief model intervention. *The Journal of Asthma, 24*(4), 199-206.
Jones, P. K., Jones, S. L., & Katz, J. (1987b). Improving follow-up among hypertensive patients using a health belief model intervention. *Archives of Internal Medicine, 147*(9), 1557-1560.
Joshi, M. S., & Bernard, D. B. (1999). Clinical performance improvement series: Classic CQI integrated with comprehensive disease management as a model for performance improvement. *The Joint Commission Journal on Quality Improvement, 25*(8), 383-395.
Kaplan, D. L., Rips, J. L., Clark, N. M., Evans, D., Wasilewski, Y., & Feldman, C. H. (1986). Transferring a clinic-based health education program for children with asthma to a school setting. *The Journal of School Health, 56*(7), 267-271.
Keefe, F. J., Caldwell, D. S., Baucom, D., Salley, A., Robinson, E., Timmons, K., Beaupre, P., Weisberg, J., & Helms, M. (1996). Spouse-assisted coping skills training in the management of osteoarthritic knee pain. *Arthritis Care and Research, 9*(4), 279-291.
Kotses, H., Stout, C., Wigal, J. K., Carlson, B., Creer, T. L., & Lewis, P. (1991). Individualized asthma self-management: A beginning. *The Journal of Asthma, 28*(4), 287-289.
Kowal, C. E. (1997). Improving asthma care in the outpatient setting. *Medical Interface, 10*(7), 87-89, 97.
Kropfelder, L. (1996). A case management approach to pediatric asthma. *Pediatric Nursing, 22*(4), 291-295.
La Forge, R., & Thomas, T. (1996). Outpatient management of lipid disorders. *The Journal of Cardiovascular Nursing, 11*(1), 39-53.
Lasater, M. (1996). The effect of a nurse-managed CHF clinic on patient readmission and length of stay. *Home Healthcare Nurse, 14*(5), 351-356.
Lasker, R. D. (1993). The diabetes control and complications trial: Implications for policy and practice (Editorial, comment). *New England Journal of Medicine, 329*(14), 1035-1036.
Lee, D., Johnson, R. A., Bingham, J. B., Leahy, M., Dinsmore, R. E., Goroll, A. H., Newell, J. B., Strauss, H. W., & Haber, E. (1982). Heart failure in outpatients: A randomized trial of digoxin versus placebo. *New England Journal of Medicine, 306*, 699-705.
Legorreta, A. P., Peters, A. L., Ossorio, R. C., Lopez, R. J., Jatulis, D. E., & Davidson, M. B. (1996). Effect of a comprehensive nurse-managed diabetes program: An HMO prospective study. *American Journal of Managed Care, 2*, 1024-1030.
Legorreta, A. P., Hasan, M. M., Peters, A. L., Pelletier, K. R., & Leung, K. M. (1997). An intervention for enhancing compliance with screening recommendations for diabetic retinopathy: A bicoastal experience. *Diabetes Care, 20*(4), 520-523.

Lewis, M. A., de la Sota, A., Rachelefsky, G., Lewis, C. E., Quinones, H., & Richards, W. (1987). ACT-asthma control y tratamiento para niños: A progress report. *Health Education Quarterly, 14*(3), 281-290.

Lewis, C. E., Rachelefsky, G., Lewis, M. A., de la Sota, A., & Kaplan, M. (1984). A randomized trial of ACT (asthma care training) for kids. *Pediatrics, 74*(4), 478-486.

Lewis, M. A., Rachelefsky, G., Lewis, C. E., Leake, B., & Richards, W. (1994). The termination of a randomized clinical trial for poor Hispanic children. *Archives of Pediatric & Adolescent Medicine, 148*(4), 364-367.

Lindroth, Y., Bauman, A., Barnes, C., McCredie, M., & Brooks, P. M. (1989). A controlled evaluation of arthritis education. *British Journal of Rheumatology, 28*(1), 7-12.

Lindroth, Y., Bauman, A., Brooks, P. M., & Priestley, D. (1995). A 5-year follow-up of a controlled trial of an arthritis education programme. *British Journal of Rheumatology, 34*(7), 647-652.

Lindroth, Y., Brattstrom, M., Bellman, I., Ekestaf, G., Olofsson, Y., Strombeck, B., Stenshed, B., Wikstrom, I., Nilsson, J. A., & Wollheim, F. A. (1997). A problem-based education program for patients with rheumatoid arthritis: Evaluation after three and twelve months. *Arthritis Care and Research, 10*(5), 325-332.

Lorig, K., Feigenbaum, P., Regan, C., Ung, E., Chastain, R. L., & Holman, H. R. (1986). A comparison of lay-taught and professional-taught arthritis self-management courses. *The Journal of Rheumatology, 13*(4), 763-767.

Lorig, K., Gonzalez, V. M., Laurent, D. D., Morgan, L., & Laris, B. A. (1998). Arthritis self-management program variations: Three studies. *Arthritis Care and Research, 11*(6), 448-454.

Lorig, K., & Holman, H. R. (1989). Long-term outcomes of an arthritis self-management study: Effects of reinforcement efforts. *Social Science & Medicine, 29*(2), 221-224.

Lorig, K., & Holman, H. R. (1993). Arthritis self-management studies: A twelve-year review. *Health Education Quarterly, 20*(1), 17-28.

Lorig, K., Lubeck, D., Kraines, R. G., Seleznick, M., & Holman, H. R. (1985). Outcomes of self-help education for patients with arthritis. *Arthritis and Rheumatism, 28*(6), 680-685.

Lorig, K. R., Mazonson, P. D., & Holman, H. R. (1993). Evidence suggesting that health education for self-management in patients with chronic arthritis has sustained health benefits while reducing health care costs. *Arthritis and Rheumatism, 36*(4), 439-446.

Lorig, K., Seleznick, M., Lubeck, D., Ung, E., Chastain, R. L., & Holman, H. R. (1989). The beneficial outcomes of the arthritis self-management course are not adequately explained by behavior change. *Arthritis and Rheumatism, 32*(1), 91-95.

Lorig, K. R., Sobel, D. S., Stewart, A. L., Brown, B. W., Jr., Bandura, A., Ritter, P., Gonzalez, V. M., Laurent, D. D., & Holman, H. R. (1999). Evidence suggesting that a chronic disease self-management program can improve health status while reducing hospitalization: A randomized trial. *Medical Care, 37*(1), 5-14.

Lorish, C. D., Parker, J., & Brown, S. (1985). Effective patient education: A quasi-experiment comparing an individualized strategy with a routinized strategy. *Arthritis and Rheumatism, 28*(11), 1289-1297.

Lozano, P., & Lieu, T. A. (1999). Asthma in managed care. *Pediatric Annals, 28*(1), 74-80.

Ludwig-Beymer, P., & Greene, A. B., Jr. (1999). Advocate Health Care's approach to adult asthma. *Chest, 116*(4, Suppl 1), 206S-207S.

Maiman, L. A., Green, L. W., Gibson, G., & MacKenzie, E. J. (1979). Education for self-treatment by adult asthmatics. *Journal of the American Medical Association, 241*(18), 1919-1922.

Mandle, C. L., Jacobs, S. C., Arcari, P., & Domar, A. D. (1996). The efficacy of relaxation response interventions with adult patients: A review of the literature. *Journal of Cardiovascular Nursing, 10,* 4-26.

Martin, T. L., Selby, J. V., & Zhang, D. (1995). Physician and patient prevention practices in NIDDM in a large urban managed-care organization. *Diabetes Care, 18*(8), 1124-1132.

Mazze, R. S., Bergenstal, R., & Ginsberg, B. (1995). Intensified diabetes management: Lessons from the diabetes control and complications trial. *International Journal of Clinical Pharmacology and Therapeutics, 33*(1), 43-51.

Mazze, R. S., Etzwiler, D. D., Strock, E., Peterson, K., McClave, C. R., Meszaros, J. F., Leigh, C., Owens, L. W., Deeb, L. C., & Peterson, A. (1994). Staged diabetes management: Toward an integrated model of diabetes care. *Diabetes Care, 17*(Suppl 1), 56-66.

Mazzuca, S. A., Brandt, K. D., Katz, B. P., Chambers, M., Byrd, D., & Hanna, M. (1997). Effects of self-care education on the health status of inner-city patients with osteoarthritis of the knee. *Arthritis and Rheumatism, 40*(8), 1466-1474.

Mazzuca, S. A., Moorman, N. H., Wheeler, M. L., Norton, J. A., Fineberg, N. S., Vinicor, F., Cohen, S. J., & Clark, C. M., Jr. (1986). The diabetes education study: A controlled trial of the effects of diabetes patient education. *Diabetes Care, 9*(1), 1-10.

McCulloch, D. K., Glasgow, R. E., Hampson, S. E., & Wagner, E. (1994). A systematic approach to diabetes management in the post-DCCT era. *Diabetes Care, 17*(7), 765-769.

McIntyre, K. M. (1995). Medicolegal implications of consensus statements. *Chest, 108*(4 Suppl), 502S-505S.

McNabb, W. L., Quinn, M. T., Murphy, D. M., Thorp, F. K., & Cook, S. (1994). Increasing children's responsibility for diabetes self-care: The in-control study. *The Diabetes Educator, 20*(2), 121-124.

McNabb, W. L., Quinn, M. T., & Rosing, I. (1993). Weight loss program for inner-city black women with non-insulin-dependent diabetes mellitus: PATHWAYS. *Journal of the American Dietetic Association, 93*(1)), 75-77.

McNabb, W. L., Wilson-Pessano, S. R., Hughes, G. W., & Scamagas, P. (1985). Self-management education of children with asthma: AIR WISE. *American Journal of Public Health, 75*(10), 1219-1220.

Moe, E. L., Eisenberg, J. D., Vollmer, W. M., Wall, M. A., Stevens, V. J., & Hollis, J. F. (1992). Implementation of "Open Airways" as an educational intervention for children with asthma in an HMO. *Journal of Pediatric Health Care, 6*(5 Part 1), 251-255.

Mullen, P. D., Laville, E. A., Biddle, A. K., & Lorig, K. (1987). Efficacy of psychoeducational interventions on pain, depression, and disability in people with arthritis: A meta-analysis. *The Journal of Rheumatology, 14* (Suppl 15), 33-39.

National Asthma Education and Prevention (NAEP) Program. (1997). *Expert panel report II: Guidelines for the diagnosis and management of asthma.* Bethesda, MD: National Institute of Health.

Neuberger, G. B., Smith, K. V., Black, S. O., & Hassanein, R. (1993). Promoting self-care in clients with arthritis. *Arthritis Care and Research, 6*(3), 141-148.

O'Brien, K. P. (1997). Asthma in the managed care setting. *Current Opinion in Pulmonary Medicine, 3*(1), 56-60.

O'Connor, P. J., & Pronk, N. P. (1998). Integrating population health concepts, clinical guidelines, and ambulatory medical systems to improve diabetes care. *Journal of Ambulatory Care Management, 21*(1), 67-73.

O'Connor, P. J., Quiter, E. S., Rush, W. A., Wiest, M., Meland, J. T., & Ryu, S. (1999). Impact of hypertension guideline implementation on blood pressure control and drug use in primary care clinics. *The Joint Commission Journal on Quality Improvement, 25*(2), 68-77.

O'Connor, P. J., Rush, W. A., Peterson, J., Morben, P., Cherney, L., Keogh, C., & Lasch, S. (1996). Continuous quality improvement can improve glycemic control for HMO patients with diabetes. *Archives of Family Medicine, 5*(9), 502-506.

O'Leary, A., Shoor, S., Lorig, K., & Holman, H. R. (1988). A cognitive-behavioral treatment for rheumatoid arthritis. *Health Psychology, 7*(6), 527-544.

Packer, M., Bristow, M. R., Cohn, J. N., Colucci, W. S., Fowler, M. B., Gilbert, E. M., & Shusterman, N. H. (1996). The effect of carvedilol on morbidity and mortality in patients with chronic heart failure. *New England Journal of Medicine, 334*(21), 1349-1355.

Packer, M., Gheorghiade, M., Young, J. B., Costantini, P. J., Adams, K. F., Cody, R. J., Smith, L. K., Van Voorhees, L., Gourley, L. A., & Jolly, M. K. (1993). Withdrawal of digoxin from patients with chronic heart failure treated with angiotensin-converting-enzyme inhibitors: RADIANCE Study. *New England Journal of Medicine, 329*(1), 1-7.

Parker, J. C., Frank, R. G., Beck, N. C., Smarr, K. L., Buescher, K. L., Phillips, L. R., Smith, E. I., Anderson, S. K., & Walker, S. E. (1988). Pain management in rheumatoid arthritis patients: A cognitive-behavioral approach. *Arthritis and Rheumatism, 31*(5), 593-601.

Parmley, W. W. (1998). Evolution of angiotensin-converting enzyme inhibition in hypertension, heart failure, and vascular protection. *The American Journal of Medicine, 105*(1A), 27S-31S.

Paul, S. (1997). Implementing an outpatient congestive heart failure clinic: The nurse practitioner role. *Heart Lung, 26*(6), 486-491.

Peters, A. L., & Davidson, M. B. (1998). Application of a diabetes managed care program: The feasibility of using nurses and a computer system to provide effective care. *Diabetes Care, 21*(7), 1037-1043.

Peters, A. L., Davidson, M. B., & Ossorio, R. C. (1995). Management of patients with diabetes by nurses with support of subspecialists. *HMO Practice, 9*(1), 8-13.

Peters, A. L., Legorreta, A. P., Ossorio, R. C., & Davidson, M. B. (1996). Quality of outpatient care provided to diabetic patients: A health maintenance organization experience. *Diabetes Care, 19*(6), 601-606.

Pfeffer, M. A., Braunwald, E., Moye, L. A., Basta, L., Brown, E. J., Jr., Cuddy, T. E., Davis, B. R., Geltman, E. M., Goldman, S., & Flaker, G. C. (1992). Effect of captopril on mortality and morbidity in patients with left ventricular dysfunction after myocardial infarction: Results of the survival and ventricular enlargement trial. *New England Journal of Medicine, 327*(10), 669-677.

Pheley, A. M., Terry, P., Pietz, L., Fowles, J., McCoy, C. E., & Smith, H. (1995). Evaluation of a nurse-based hypertension management program: Screening, management, and outcomes. *The Journal of Cardiovascular Nursing, 9*(2), 54-61.

Plaut, T. F., Howell, T., Walsh, S., Pastor, M., & Jones, T. (1996). A systems approach to asthma care. *Managed Care Quarterly, 4*(3), 6-18.

Pugh, L. C., Tringali, R. A., Boehmer, J., Blaha, C., Kruger, N. R., Capauna, T. A., Bryan, Y., Robinson, J., Belmont, D., Young, M., & Xie, S. (1999). Partners in care: A model of collaboration. *Holistic Nursing Practice, 13*(2), 61-65.

Rich, M. W. (1999). Heart failure disease management: A critical review. *Journal of Cardiac Failure, 5*(1), 64-75.

Rich, M. W., Beckham, V., Wittenberg, C., Leven, C. L., Freedland, K. E., & Carney, R. M. (1995). A multidisciplinary intervention to prevent the readmission of elderly patients with congestive heart failure. *New England Journal of Medicine, 333*(18), 1190-1195.

Rich, M. W., Gray, D. B., Beckham, V., Wittenberg, C., & Luther, P. (1996). Effect of a multidisciplinary intervention on medication compliance in elderly patients with congestive heart failure. *The American Journal of Medicine, 101,* 270-276.

Rich, M. W., Vinson, J. M., Sperry, J. C., Shah, A. S., Spinner, L. R., Chung, M. K., & Davila-Roman, V. (1993). Prevention of readmission in elderly patients with congestive heart failure: Results of a prospective, randomized pilot study. *Journal of General Internal Medicine, 8*(11), 585-590.

Rippey, R. M., Bill, D., Abeles, M., Day, J., Downing, D. S., Pfeiffer, C. A., Thal, S. E., & Wetstone, S. L. (1987). Computer-based patient education for older persons with osteoarthritis. *Arthritis and Rheumatism, 30*(8), 932-935.

Rosenstein, A. H. (1997). Using information management to implement a clinical resource management program. *The Joint Commission Journal on Quality Improvement, 23*(12), 653-666.

Rosenstock, I. M. (1985). Understanding and enhancing patient compliance with diabetic regimens. *Diabetes Care, 8*(6), 610-616.

Rubin, R. J., Dietrich, K. A., & Hawk, A. D. (1998). Clinical and economic impact of implementing a comprehensive diabetes management program in managed care. *Journal of Clinical Endocrinology and Metabolism, 83*(8), 2635-2642.

Sadur C. N., Moline, N., Costa, M., Mendlowitz, D., Roller, S., Watson, R., Swain, S. E., Selby, J. V., & Javorski, W. C. (1999). Diabetes management in a health maintenance organization. *Diabetes Care, 22,* 2011-2017.

Schned, E. S., Doyle, M. A., Glickstein, S. L., Schousboe, J. T., Reinertsen, J. L., Baglioni, A. J., & Tolson, T. F. (1995). Team managed outpatient care for early onset chronic inflammatory arthritis. *The Journal of Rheumatology, 22*(6), 1141-1148.

Schultz, J. F., & Sheps, S. G. (1994). Management of patients with hypertension: A hypertension clinic model. *Mayo Clinic Proceedings, 69*(10), 997-999.

Seabrook, G. R., Karp, D., Schmitt, D. D., Bandyk, D. F., & Towne, J. B. (1990). An outpatient anticoagulation protocol managed by a vascular nurse-clinician. *American Journal of Surgery, 160*(5), 501-505.

Self, T., & Nolan, S. (1997). Long-term management of asthma: How to improve outcomes. *American Journal of Managed Care, 3*(9), 1425-1438.

Shah, N. B., Der, E., Ruggerio, C., Heidenreich, P. A., & Massie, B. M. (1998). Prevention of hospitalizations for heart failure with an interactive home monitoring program. *American Heart Journal, 135*(3), 373-378.

Shields, M. C., Griffin, K. W., & McNabb, W. L. (1990). The effect of a patient education program on emergency room use for inner-city children with asthma. *American Journal of Public Health, 80*(1), 36-38.

Sigurd, B., Olesen, K. H., & Wennevold, A. (1975). The supra-additive natriuretic effect addition of bendroflumethiazide and bumetanide in congestive heart failure: Permutation trial tests in patients in long-term treatment with bumetanide. *American Heart Journal, 89*(2), 163-170.

Singer, D. L. (1995). A self-management approach to diabetes care: The Harvard Community Health Plan experience. *Health Care Innovations, 5*(5), 17-24.

Smith, L. E., Fabbri, S. A., Pai, R., Ferry, D., & Heywood, J. T. (1997). Symptomatic improvement and reduced hospitalization for patients attending a cardiomyopathy clinic. *Clinical Cardiology, 20*(11), 949-954.

Smith, S. A., Murphy, M. E., Huschka, T. R., Dinneen, S. F., Gorman, C. A., Zimmerman, B. R., Rizza, R. A., & Naessens, J. M. (1998). Impact of a diabetes electronic management system on the care of patients seen in a subspecialty diabetes clinic. *Diabetes Care, 21*(6), 972-976.

Snyder, S. E., Winder, J. A., & Creer, T. J. (1987). Development and evaluation of an adult asthma self-management program: Wheezers Anonymous. *The Journal of Asthma, 24*(3), 153-158.

Solberg, L. I., Reger, L. A., Pearson, T. L., Cherney, L. M., O'Connor, P. J., Freemen, S. L., Lasch, S. L., & Bishop, D. B. (1997). Using continuous quality improvement to improve diabetes care in populations: The IDEAL model. Improving care for diabetics through empowerment active collaboration and leadership. *The Joint Commission Journal on Quality Improvement, 23*(11), 581-592.

The SOLVD Investigators. (1991). Effect of analapril on survival in patients with reduced left ventricular ejection fraction. *New England Journal of Medicine, 325,* 293-302.

The SOLVD Investigators. (1992). Effect of enalapril on mortality and the development of heart failure in asymptomatic patients with reduced left ventricular ejection fractions. *New England Journal of Medicine, 327,* 685-691.

Stevens, M. A. & Weiss-Harrison, A. (1993). A program for children with asthma. *HMO Practice, 7*(2), 91-93.

Strauss, G. D., Spiegel, J. S., Daniels, M., Spiegel, T., Landsverk, J., Roy-Byrne, P., Edelstein, C., Ehlhardt, J., Falke, R., & Hindin, L. (1986). Group therapies for rheumatoid arthritis: A controlled study of two approaches. *Arthritis and Rheumatism, 29*(10), 1203-1209.

Sullivan, M. J., & Hawthorne, M. H. (1996). Nonpharmacologic interventions in the treatment of heart failure. *The Journal of Cardiovascular Nursing, 10*(2), 47-57.

Sullivan, S., Elixhauser, A., Buist, A. S., Luce, B. R., Eisenberg, J., & Weiss, K. B. (1996). National Asthma Education and Prevention Program working group report on the cost effectiveness of asthma care. *American Journal of Respiratory and Critical Care Medicine, 154*(3, Part 2), S84-S95.

Taggart, V. S., Zuckerman, A. E., Lucas, S., Acty-Lindsey, A., & Bellanti, J. A. (1987). Adapting a self-management education program for asthma for use in an outpatient clinic. *Annals of Allergy, 58*(3), 173-178.

Taggart, V. S., Zuckerman, A. E., Sly, R. M., Steinmueller, C., Newman, G., O'Brien, R. W., Schneider, S., & Bellanti, J. A. (1991). You can control asthma: Evaluation of an asthma education program for hospitalized inner-city children. *Patient Education and Counseling, 17*(1), 35-47.

Terry, K. (1997). Where disease management is paying off. *Medical Economics, 74*(14), 62-62.

Topol, E. J., Traill, T. A., & Fortuin, N. J. (1985). Hypertensive hypertrophic cardiomyopathy of the elderly. *New England Journal of Medicine, 312*(5), 277-283.

Topp, R., Tucker, D., & Weber, C. (1998). Effect of a clinical case manager/clinical nurse specialist on patients hospitalized with congestive heart failure. *Nursing Case Management, 3*(4), 140-145.

Trubitt, M. J. (1999). United HealthCare of Illinois: Working to improve asthma care. *Chest, 116*(4 Suppl 1), 208S-209S.

Urden, L. D. (1998). Heart failure collaborative care: An integrated partnership to manage quality and outcomes. *Outcomes Management for Nursing Practice, 2*(2), 64-70.
Venner, G. H., & Seelbinder, J. S. (1996). Team management of congestive heart failure across the continuum. *The Journal of Cardiovascular Nursing, 10*(2), 71-84.
Waagstein, F., Bristow, M. R., Swedberg, K., Camerini, F., Fowler, M. B., Silver, M. A., Gilbert, E. M., Johnson, M. R., Goss, F. G., & Hjalmarson, A. (1993). Beneficial effects of metoprolol in idiopathic dilated cardiomyopathy. *Lancet, 342,* 1441-1446.
Wagner, E. H. (1995). Population-based management of diabetes care. *Patient Education and Counseling, 26*(1-3), 225-230.
Wagner, E. H. (1996). The promise and performance of HMOs in improving outcomes in older adults. *Journal of the American Geriatric Society, 44*(10), 1251-1257.
Wagner, E. H. (1997). Managed care and chronic illness: Health services research needs. *Health Services Research, 32*(5), 702-714.
Wagner, E. H., Austin, B. T., & Von Korff, M. (1996). Organizing care for patients with chronic illness. *Milbank Quarterly, 74*(4), 511-544.
Weinberger, M., Oddone, E. Z., & Henderson, W. G. (1996). Does increased access to primary care reduce hospital readmissions? *New England Journal of Medicine, 334*(22), 1441-1447.
West, J. A., Miller, N. H., Parker, K. M., Senneca, D., Ghandour, G., Clark, M., Greenwald, G., Heller, R. S., Fowler, M. B., & DeBusk, R. F. (1997). A comprehensive management system for heart failure improves clinical outcomes and reduces medical resource utilization. *The American Journal of Cardiology, 79*(1), 58-63.
Wetstone, S. L., Sheehan, T. J., Votaw, R. G., Peterson, M. G., & Rothfield, N. (1985). Evaluation of a computer-based education lesson for patients with rheumatoid arthritis. *The Journal of Rheumatology* 12(5), 907-912.
Whight, C., Morgan, T., Carney, S., & Wilson, M. (1974). Diuretics, cardiac failure, and potassium depletion: A rational approach. *The Medical Journal of Australia, 2*(23), 831-833.
Wilkes, R. M, Dukes, K. R., Feagles, L. L., Leong, D., & Allen, G. L. (1999). Kaiser Permanente's approach to congestive heart failure in south San Francisco. *Journal of Critical Outcomes Management, 6*(5), 37-40.
Wilson, S. R., Latini, D., Starr, N. J., Fish, L., Loes, L. M., Page, A., & Kubic, P. (1996). Education of parents of infants and very young children with asthma: A developmental evaluation of the Wee Wheezers program. *The Journal of Asthma, 33*(4), 239-254. (Published erratum appears in *The Journal of Asthma,* 34[3], 261; 1997)
Wilson, S. R., Scamagas, P., German, D. F., Hughes, G. W., Lulla, S., Coss, S., Chardon, L., Thomas, R. G., Starr-Schneidkraut, N., & Stancavage, F. B. (1993). A controlled trial of two forms of self-management education for adults with asthma. *The American Journal of Medicine, 94*(6), 564-576.
Wilson, S. R., Scamagas, P., Grado, J., Norgaard, L., Starr, N. J., Eaton, S., & Pomaville, K. (1998). The Fresno Asthma Project: A model intervention to control asthma in multiethnic, low-income, inner-city communities. *Health, Education, & Behavior, 25*(1), 79-98.
Wilson-Pessano, S. R., & McNabb, W. L. (1985). The role of patient education in the management of childhood asthma. *Preventive Medicine, 14*(6), 670-687.
Wilson-Pessano, S. R., Scamagas, P., Arsham, G. M., Chardon, L., Coss, S., German, D. F., & Hughes, G. W. (1987). An evaluation of approaches to asthma self-management education for adults: The AIR/Kaiser-Permanente Study. *Health Education Quarterly, 14*(3), 333-343.

Wilt, V. M., Gums, J. G., Ahmed, O. I., & Moore, L. M. (1995). Outcome analysis of a pharmacist-managed anticoagulation service. *Pharmacotherapy, 15*(6), 732-739.

Young, J. B., Gheorghiade, M., Uretsky, B. F., Patterson, J. H., & Adams, K. F., Jr. (1998). Superiority of "triple" drug therapies in heart failure: Insights from the PROVED and RADIANCE trials. *Journal of the American College of Cardiology, 32*, 686-692.

Young, L. D., Bradley, L. A., & Turner, R. A. (1995). Decreases in health care resource utilization in patients with rheumatoid arthritis following a cognitive behavioral intervention. *Biofeedback and Self-Regulation, 20*(3), 259-268.

Zeiger, R. S., Heller, S., Mellon, M. H., Wald, J., Falkoff, R., & Schatz, M. (1991). Facilitated referral to asthma specialist reduces relapses in asthma emergency room visits. *The Journal of Allergy and Clinical Immunology, 87*(6), 1160-1168. (Published erratum appears in *The Journal of Allergy and Clinical Immunology, 90*[2], 278; 1992)

7 Conclusions and Future Research Directions

In this final chapter, we make some overall observations that build on the previous chapters and then speculate on how changes in the future of managed care could raise new research questions relating to managed care and chronic illness.

Observations on Existing Research

As we noted in Chapters 3 through 6, there are surprisingly few rigorous studies on most topics relating to managed care and people with chronic illness. Critiques and summaries of the existing literature are found at the end of each chapter, and we will not repeat those discussions in this chapter. In most cases, we argued for more research. However, we believe that better research is also needed. And, in some cases, we believe that researchers need to expand the organizational settings for their research efforts and adopt new paradigms to address new research topics.

Improving the quality of research. Improving the quality of research in this area, although important, will not be easy. In part, this relates to two major obstacles that are inherent in doing research that focuses on patients with chronic as opposed to acute illnesses. The first obstacle is that chronic illnesses, by their nature, play out over extended time periods—they are "lived with" illnesses—and this raises several issues for researchers. Patients may experience periods when the progression of the illness appears halted and, for some illnesses, they may experience periods of acute symptoms. However, the general trajectory of these illnesses is typically downward. Initiatives implemented by managed care organizations (MCOs) may alter the slope of this trajectory and possibly minimize the number and depth of acute episodes experienced by patients, but they will not accomplish a cure.

This poses a significant problem for researchers: how to accurately measure the impact of MCO initiatives on patient outcomes and on costs. The group of patients treated under an initiative must be followed for a significant period of time and contrasted to an appropriate control group, tracked over the same time period. This means that, first, both the initiative and the control group must, at the beginning of the study, contain a substantial number of participants, because attrition from the study is often an issue over extended follow-up periods. This is particularly problematic for the evaluation of an initiative carried out within a single MCO, because attrition may occur not only because of death or "study fatigue" but also because patients choose voluntarily to switch health plans or are forced to switch due to decisions on the part of their employers. Depending on the type of illness, an MCO may need substantial enrollment to generate the number of participants required for the study. Or, the study design may need to involve multiple MCOs, all of whom agree to implement an initiative of the same design over the same time period. A multiple MCO study typically is very difficult to mount and sustain over time, but a single MCO study may not yield enough participants to assess the effectiveness of the intervention. In either case, a consequence of the need to enroll substantial numbers of study participants, and track them over a significant period of time, is that the study is likely to be expensive. This makes it difficult for MCOs to mount credible studies using internal resources and limits the potential external sources of funding.

The need to track participants over an extended time period to detect shifts in their illness trajectories can also make the recruitment of MCOs as study participants difficult. For many MCOs, survival is a year-to-year question. They may be unable or unwilling to commit to an extended research time frame. Also, they may question the likely relevance to them of study findings in an industry where dramatic new pharmaceutical advances are occurring on a regular basis. They may be more interested in evaluating initiatives that hold the promise of improved bottom lines in the short term rather than improved patient outcomes in the long run.

There is a second problem facing researchers that also relates to the nature of chronic illness: Patients, especially elderly patients, often suffer from multiple chronic illnesses simultaneously. Although some MCO initiatives, particularly those that focus on managing the care of high-cost patients, are designed to address this phenomenon, many single-illness initiatives are not. The major implication of this for research is that it makes it more difficult to detect initiative outcomes—favorable or unfavorable. For a patient with multiple illnesses, changes in the trajectory of health status caused by an MCO initiative may be masked or muted by the presence of symptoms associated with the patient's other conditions. Thus, sensitive measures are needed to detect changes in patient outcomes related to the initiative. Unfortunately, the measures used in most published studies of MCO chronic illness initiatives were generally not designed with this in mind. Often, they are measures used in studies of acute-care processes and some are ill-suited to evaluations of chronic illness initiatives.

Expanding the settings for research. A second general observation about the existing literature is that much of the research pertaining to managed care initiatives in the treatment of chronic illness has been carried out in a relatively small number of organizations. In particular, the organizations that are most frequently studied include Kaiser of Northern California, Group Health of Puget Sound, and HealthPartners in Minneapolis/St. Paul, Minnesota. The fact that these organizations are often settings for this type of research is understandable. They have played leadership roles in the managed care industry in developing and implementing treatment initiatives for chronic illness and therefore are obvious laboratories for evaluating the effectiveness of these initiatives.

Also, they have internal expertise in evaluation research that facilitates evaluation efforts. Much of what is known about the treatment of chronic illnesses in managed care settings is a direct consequence of the willingness of these MCOs to subject their own efforts to research scrutiny.

Clearly, the limited number and types of managed-care organizational settings in which research relating to chronic illness treatment has been carried out raise questions of generalizability of findings. The most popular types of MCOs, measured by enrollment and number, are more loosely integrated than the organizations used as traditional sites for research. Preferred provider organizations (PPOs) and independent physician association (IPA)-model health maintenance organizations (HMOs) enroll a substantial proportion of the employed population. Because these organizations are characterized by large, geographically dispersed provider networks, coordination of care for people with chronic illnesses is likely to be difficult. The problem becomes more complex for organizations or products that permit patients to go "out of network" at the point of service. In these situations, chronic-care initiatives might revolve around system-level information systems that support providers in the tracking of patient service use and health outcomes and help patients in their self-management efforts. However, very little is known about whether and how these types of MCOs attempt to manage care for people with chronic illness and if their initiatives are effective.

To expand our knowledge, it would be useful to expand the number and types of research settings to include these and other types of managed care settings, including organizations that focus on the management of specific diseases. Unfortunately, any attempt to generate research findings that are more representative of managed care in general will confront two obstacles. First, in a competitive market environment, there may be no compelling reason for MCOs to participate in evaluations of their chronic illness management efforts. Indeed, there is a risk involved, because the evaluation findings could be negative and used by competitors to discredit the MCO. Perhaps more important, the generalizability of the evaluation results would continue to be limited, due to possible volunteer bias. That is, MCOs of any type that agree to be evaluated by unbiased researchers using a rigorous research design might do so because they expect favorable outcomes. These outcomes would not necessarily be achievable in an average MCO. This means that published research findings related to chronic illness initiatives in MCOs could present a misleading, overly favorable impression of effectiveness.

Expanding the research focus. In this book, we have organized our discussion around topics addressed in the existing literature. A critical assessment of that literature, however, calls for identification of important areas of research that are largely missing from the published body of work relating to managed care and chronic illness. In our opinion, the existing literature could be enhanced in very important ways by greater attention to organizational issues and how they affect the design, implementation, sustainability, and ultimate success of chronic illness management programs implemented in MCOs. Relatively little research attention has been directed at decision making within MCOs regarding the structure of care for people with chronic illness and the support given to new chronic-care initiatives. Organizational issues around chronic care can be quite complex because implementation of new initiatives may require restructuring care-delivery processes in fundamental ways, affect a large number of internal organizational stakeholders, consume significant organizational resources, and raise relatively difficult managerial issues. Understanding the role of organizational facilitators and constraints would perhaps clarify why many well-documented and carefully evaluated chronic illness management initiatives have never progressed beyond the pilot stage to become part of "usual care" in MCOs.

There has been even less attention given to identifying and understanding the factors that can lead MCOs to cut back or eliminate functioning chronic care management programs that appear to have been successful. It is particularly striking when organizations such as Lovelace and the University of Pennsylvania, which have been nationally recognized advocates for innovative chronic illness management initiatives, withdraw or significantly reduce their support. The reduction of support for chronic illness management models on the part of organizations that have previously been strong advocates has the potential to discourage innovation among other MCOs. It raises questions that could be addressed through carefully designed and executed qualitative research projects that document the circumstances contributing to these decisions and dissect the organizational decision-making processes employed.

Research Challenges for the Future

The questions that future researchers will be called on to address that relate to managed care and chronic illness are likely to differ from the questions addressed by the research studies summarized in this book. In our opinion, three factors are likely to be the most important in influencing the nature of the questions addressed by future researchers: the development of new pharmaceuticals for the treatment of different chronic illnesses; the growth in availability and use of information technologies, such as the Internet, for patient self-management and clinician management; and the restructuring of the employer role in the health insurance market.

New pharmaceuticals. Over the past 5 years, numerous new drugs have become available for use by patients with chronic illnesses. Some of these drugs have addressed primarily symptom alleviation, but others have shown promise in retarding the progression of specific chronic illnesses. The pace of drug development appears to be accelerating, in part due to the aging of the population, which increases the number of individuals with chronic illnesses and therefore expands the potential market for new drugs. Pharmaceutical companies have increasingly directed their advertising at patients (Hollon, 1999; Holmer, 1999). Presumably, they hope that patients will pressure their physicians to argue for including these drugs on MCO formularies. How will MCOs respond to these new opportunities for drug treatment of chronic illnesses? As medications are added to formularies, how will they become incorporated in treatment regimes? To what degree will MCOs increase patient cost-sharing to compensate for increased overall treatment costs? Or, will overall costs decline, as effective drug therapy reduces the probability of disease flare-up and the subsequent need for acute care? How will potentially complicated poly-pharmacy situations be managed within MCOs? How will MCO strategies to manage pharmaceutical costs for people with chronic illnesses affect drug use, costs, and patient outcomes? What strategies will be the most cost-effective? These sorts of questions are, of course, relevant in the present environment and have been addressed by some researchers. But, we believe they will receive much more research attention in the future.

Use of information technologies. The impact of new information technology, and particularly the Internet, on consumers and businesses has been felt in all sectors of the economy, including health care. Experts predict that effects to date will seem minimal in comparison to future impacts, as technological breakthroughs continue, costs decline, and the use of technologies such as the Internet spreads from early adopters to the general population. Some of the implications for chronic illness management can already be observed. Chat rooms bring together, anonymously, people with similar illnesses for mutual support and exchange of information regarding pharmaceuticals and treatment regimes. In addition, patients can access a very large number of different Web sites that provide them with information about their diseases and possible treatment approaches (Goldsmith, 2000). Whereas some of these sites are intended to provide impartial assessments, others are maintained for the purpose of selling particular products that may or may not be effective in improving patient health. The electronic transmission of medical records is becoming increasingly common, making better coordination of treatment possible, at least in theory (Dunbrack, 2000). Also, more sophisticated information systems are being developed to assist clinicians in monitoring patient treatment and health outcomes (Goldstein, 2000). How will MCOs incorporate new developments in information technology in the treatment of chronic illness? How will they respond to the demands of the empowered patient with chronic illness? To what extent, and how quickly, will the potential for these new technologies to improve patient care be realized, given the cost of adoption and the limited discretionary funding available to many MCOs? Will there be any measurable effect on the health of chronically ill patients in MCOs?

Restructuring of the employer role. Recent double-digit health insurance-premium increases are causing employers to reexamine their traditional role as employee agents in the purchase of health insurance (Landers, 2000). The confidence of employers in the ability of existing models for managed care to control costs, while at the same time meeting employee demands for a broad choice of providers and easy access to the physicians of their choice, has been tested. At least some employers are now examining new approaches to health care purchasing that would reduce their intermediary agent role and disconnect their contribution toward premiums from rates of increase in premiums. These approaches are also often designed to reduce employer legal liability related to employee experience in managed care plans offered as health benefits by the employer. Under what have been labeled *defined contribution* strategies, employers would contribute a fixed dollar amount toward employee health insurance, with the employee assuming primary responsibility for the purchase of that insurance (Reese, 2000; Trude & Ginsburg, 2000). Under one scenario, employees would seek out insurance options that met their individual needs, possibly using the Internet to search across available plans. They would essentially enter the present individual insurance market armed with a fixed amount of dollars provided by their employer. Under a more unconventional scenario, employees would essentially create their own provider network and insurance coverage using Internet broker organizations, with employers again contributing a fixed dollar amount toward the final price (Parente, 2000).

The extent to which employers will adopt any type of defined-contribution approach, or otherwise reduce their presence as employee agents in the health insurance market, is difficult to predict. If they do move in this direction, the implications for employees or their dependents with chronic illnesses will vary depending on the specific strategy adopted by the employer. For instance, if the employer does not risk-adjust the defined contribution, people with chronic illness will pay a much larger portion of their health insurance premiums than they do at present. How will this affect the types of managed care plans they select? Will they choose lower cost but more tightly managed plans in an attempt to minimize the financial impact of this change? How will this affect their access to care and use of services? Their health status over time? If employers offer their employees the option of essentially constructing their own networks and determining their own co-payments and deductibles, how will employees with chronic illnesses respond? Which providers will they include in their networks? What factors will be important in those decisions? How will they trade off their desire for access and low copayments with the higher premiums that would likely result? How will MCOs respond to this new health insurance-purchasing environment? What products would evolve in response to the demands of people with chronic illnesses? What will be the impact of new insurance arrangements and a reduced employer role in the health insurance market on the health of people with chronic illnesses?

In summary, we believe that managed care will exist in some form in the near future, although it will continue to reshape itself in response to public policy, employer decisions, and ongoing innovation in pharmaceuticals and in information technology. The number of people with chronic illnesses will continue to increase, both absolutely and as a percentage of the population. Therefore, understanding how different aspects of managed care affect people with chronic illnesses will continue to be an important research area; in fact, it will grow in importance. The existing research provides a foundation for addressing these developing issues, but that foundation is neither particularly broad or deep. This is because the challenges that researchers face in carrying out rigorous research in this area are formidable and are likely to remain so in the future.

References

Dunbrack, L. (2000, March/April). E-disease management: The technology solution. *Healthplan*, pp. 65-68.
Goldsmith, J. (2000). How will the Internet change our health system? *Health Affairs, 19*(1), 48-156.
Goldstein, D. (2000). The e-healthcare cyber tsunami. *Managed Care Quarterly, 8*(3), 9-14.
Hollon, M. F. (1999). Direct-to-consumer marketing of prescription drugs: Creating consumer demand. *Journal of the American Medical Association, 281*(4), 382-384.
Holmer, A. F. (1999). Direct-to-consumer prescription drug advertising builds bridges between patients and physicians. *Journal of the American Medical Association, 281*(4), 380-382.
Landers, S. (2000, August 14). Employers mull cash in lieu of health insurance for workers. *American Medical News*, pp. 1-3.
Parente, S. (2000). Beyond the hype: A taxonomy of e-health business models. *Health Affairs, 19*(6), 1-14.
Reese, S. (2000, March). New concepts in health benefits: Defined contribution. *Business and Health*, pp. 31-33.

Trude, S., & Ginsburg, P. (2000, October). *Are defined contributions a new direction for employer sponsored coverage?* (Issue Brief No. 32). Washington, DC: Center for Studying Health System Change.

Index

Abington Memorial Hospital, 222
Abourizk, N. N., 122, 127, 130, 138
Abraham, W. T., 16
Academic journals, 10
Accreditation, 31, 67, 91
ACE inhibitors, 115, 138, 141, 144, 214, 223
Acty-Lindsey, A., 133
Acute care, 22-23
Acute illness, 3
Adams, K. F., Jr., 141
Administrative and medical records data. *See* Chronic illness management, use of administrative and medical records data
Adult Diabetes Education Program and Training (ADEPT), 190
Adult Outpatient Asthma Education Project, 195
Advertising, 260
Advocate Health Care, 211
Agency for Health Care Policy (AHCPR), 138, 141, 213
AIR POWER, 133, 135, 196
AIR WISE, 133, 135, 196, 200
Alexander, M., 94, 109
Alexander, W. A., 154, 237
Allen, G. L., 16, 138

Allen, H., 55
Allen, S. M., 22
Alt, K. J., 163
Amato, M. G., 150
American Diabetes Association (ADA), 91, 114, 125, 173, 183
American Heart Association, 16
American Institutes of Research (AIR), 210
Amin, S. P., 106
Anderson, J., 154, 161, 237
Anderson, R. M., 122
Ankylosing spondylitis, 155
Anticoagulation Monitoring Service, 234
Anticoagulation therapy, 95, 109, 147, 150, 152-153
  hospital-based interventions, 154
  memberwide interventions, 151
  nurse-managed intervention, 232
  pharmacist-managed intervention, 233-235
  program components, 158-159
  summary of studies (table), 232-235
  See also Cardiovascular disease management
Aranda, J. M., 146
Arcari, P., 141
Arnold, S. B., 141

Arthritis, 15-16
Arthritis management, 15-16
　disease management programs, 69
　health outcome indicators, 162-163
　identification of improvement
　　opportunities, 109
　intervention effectiveness studies, 155,
　　162-166
　　　components of programs, 167
　　　educational interventions, 162-
　　　　167
　　　programwide interventions,
　　　　164-166
　　　self-management, 164
　　　summary, 166
　multidisciplinary team approach, 165,
　　167, 241
　patient characteristics, HMO versus
　　fee-for-service programs, 45
　program development and
　　implementation, 79
　self-management support, 164, 240
　service utilization and outcomes,
　　MCOs versus fee-for-service, 51-52,
　　56-57
　summary of studies (table), 240-241
　vendor products, 167
Arthur, M. W., 163
Aspen Medical Group, 136, 198
Aspirin use, 13
Asthma, 4, 13
Asthma management, 14, 69, 73, 83-85
　AIR WISE, 133, 135, 196, 200
　cost-effectiveness modeling, 109
　cross-HMO studies, 59
　development and implementation of
　　programs, 75-76, 78
　disease programs, 69, 73
　educational interventions, 132-133, 195-
　　201, 204, 205, 209, 210, 211
　effective intervention implementation
　　issues, 115
　Episodes of Care, 81, 208
　high-risk populations, 28, 99-100, 108
　identification of improvement
　　opportunities, 106, 108
　inhaled anti-inflammatory medication,
　　84, 93, 115, 131-133, 195, 197, 202,
　　204
　intervention effectiveness studies, 131-
　　138
　　　clinical outcome measures, 133-
　　　　136
　　　costs, 136-137
　　　memberwide interventions, 133-
　　　　134
　　　program components (table),
　　　　139-140
　　　programwide interventions,
　　　　134-137
　　　socioeconomic/minority status
　　　　and, 137, 138
　　　summary, 137-138
　nurse case management, 203, 205
　peak-flow meters (PFMs), 115, 132, 197,
　　199
　practice guidelines, 93, 107, 131
　provider profiling, 98, 108
　quality improvement initiatives, 208-
　　209
　summary of studies (table), 195-211
　vendor products, 81, 83-86, 140
Asthma Care Training (ACT) for Kids,
　132, 135, 136, 201
Asthma Education and Primary Care
　Clinician Linkages, 208
Asthma Integrated Management (AIM),
　85
Asthma Kits, 84
Asthma Outreach Program (AOP), 205
Atlantic Medical Services, Inc., 202
Attrition, 131, 138, 151-152, 256
Aubert, R. E., 125, 130, 131, 180
Aucott, J. N., 154
Austin, A., x, xii, 23, 68, 70-72, 86, 114
Australia/New Zealand Heart Failure
　Research Collaborative Group, 141
Automated reminders, 120, 121
　anticoagulation interventions, 158
　arthritis interventions, 167
　asthma interventions, 139
　cardiovascular disease interventions,
　　160
　diabetes interventions, 128
　heart failure interventions, 148
　hypertension interventions, 156, 229
Automated medical records, 100

Baglioni, A. J., Jr., 163
Baltimore Alliance for the Prevention and Control of Hypertension and Diabetes, 117, 187, 231
Bandyk, D. F., 154
Barefoot, J., 163
Barefoot doctor program, 187, 231
Barlow, J. H., 163
Barnes, C., 163-164
Barr, D. A., 29
Barrella, P., 142, 146, 149, 222
Barstow, T. J., 141
Basler, H. D., 163
Bauman, A., 163-164
Bayliss, M. S., 48
Baystate Medical Center, 176
Beary, J. F., 141
Beauregard, K. M., 45-46
Becker, A., 132, 154, 159
Becker, D. M., 232
Beckham, V., 115
Begg, C. G., 56
Behavioral change outcomes, 153, 162, 215, 227
Behavioral Risk Factor Surveillance System (BRFSS), 46
Belardinelli, R., 141
Bellanti, J. A., 133
Benchmarking, 91-93, 105-107
Benjamin, E. M., 130, 176
Benson, H., 141
Bensussen-Walls, W., 122
Berenson, R., 24
Berenstein, A., 49, 55
Berg, C. E., 163
Bergelson, A., 82-83, 169
Bergenstal, R., 12, 82, 122
Bernard, D. B., 130, 169, 194
Best practice guidelines. *See* Chronic illness management, guidelines and care protocols
Beta blockers, 17, 141
Beth Israel Hospital, 181
Bhattacharyya, S. K., 105, 106, 107
Biddle, A. K., 162
Bigas, C., 146
Bill-Harvey, D., 164
Bilodeau, A., 15, 162
Birmann, B. M., 107

Black, S. O., 163
Blue Care Network, 190, 197
Blue Cross and Blue Shield, 195, 197
Blumethal, D., 35
Boggs, P. B., 115
Borgess Medical Care Center, 218
Boult, C., 70, 71
Boxerman, S. B., 42
Bradley, L. A., 163
Brady-Green Community Health Center, 233
Brass-Mynderse, N. J., 149, 212
Brenden, J., 23, 24
Bristow, M. R., 16, 138
Brooks, P. M., 163-164
Brosnan, J., 155
Brown, B., 56, 58, 60
Brown, E., 69
Brown, J., 96, 106
Brown, J. B., x
Brown, R. S., 57
Brown, S., 163
Brunk, S. E., 163
Brunner, C. M., 163
Buchmueller, T. C., 42
Buchner, D. A., 84, 85, 115, 133-134, 137, 140, 202
Buist, A. S., 107
Buntin, M. B., 35
Busch, A. J., 163
Bussey, H. I., 150, 154, 159, 233
Butterworth Hospital, 219

Caldwell, J. R., 29
Calfas, K. J., 163
Callahan, D., 3
Cantor, J. C., 153, 157, 225
Capitation payment arrangements, 24, 27, 28, 33-34
Caplan, A. L., 3
Cardiovascular disease, 4
Cardiovascular disease management, 13
  benchmarking, 109
  case-management program, 236
  continuous quality improvement initiative, 237
  costs and utilization, 96
  educational interventions, 225-227

intervention effectiveness studies, 147, 150-155
   behavioral outcomes, 153
   care guidelines, 150
   components of programs, 156-161
   hospital-based interventions, 153-154
   memberwide interventions, 151-152
   process of care, 153
   programwide interventions, 152-153
   study common features and limitations, 155
patient characteristics, HMO versus fee-for-service programs, 45
pharmacist-managed intervention, 233-235
quality of care guidelines, 109
risk factors, 13
summary of studies (table), 225-239
See also Anticoagulation therapy; Dyslipidemia management; Hypertension management
Carey, C., 164-167
Carnegie Mellon University, 42
Carney, M. F., 56
Carney, S., 141
Carve-out arrangements, 35, 80-81
   anticoagulation interventions, 159
   arthritis interventions, 167
   asthma interventions, 140
   cardiovascular disease interventions, 161
   diabetes interventions, 129
   heart failure interventions, 149
   hypertension interventions, 157
Case management, 68, 71
   anticoagulation intervention, 236
   cardiovascular disease interventions, 153
   congestive heart failure intervention, 219
   diabetes intervention, 188
   See also Nurse case management
Case mix, 97
Cassou, S., 43
Cave, D. G., 35

Cedars Sinai Medical Center, 182-184
Centers for Disease Control, 123, 192, 193
Cesta, T. G., 122, 127
Chernew, M., 42
Chicoye, L., 13, 114, 126, 130, 169, 189
The Childhood Asthma Project, 133
Chima, C. S., 154, 161, 169, 238
Chiquette, E., 150
Cholesterol management. *See* Cardiovascular disease management; Dyslipidemia management
Christianson, J. B., 157, 229
Chronic illness:
   defining, 3-5
   descriptions of specific illnesses, 11-17
Chronic illness management:
   at-risk populations. *See* High-risk patients or populations
   "carve-outs," 35. *See* Carve-out arrangements
   effectiveness assessment, 75
   multiple disease services, 74
   multiple morbidities, 22, 257
   physician profiling. *See* Physician profiling
   physician support for programs, 66-67
   PPO involvement, 77
   program cutback or elimination, 259
   program development and implementation, 74-79
   program implementation barriers, 71
   simulation models, 100-105
   sustainability of interventions, 170-171
   trends, 22-23
   vendor products. *See* Vendor products
   See also Arthritis management; Asthma management; Cardiovascular disease management; Congestive heart failure management; Diabetes management
Chronic illness management, effectiveness of targeted initiatives:
   arthritis, 155, 162-166
   asthma, 131-138
   cardiovascular diseases, 147, 150-155
   classification of interventions, 120-121
   common features of effective programs, 169

Index

common limitations of reviewed studies, 131, 147
congestive heart failure, 138, 141-147
definitions, 116
diabetes, 122-131
efficacy trials and, 113-114
high-risk patients and, 117-118, 137
implementation issues, 114-115
indicators, 116, 125
literature search results (table), 118
patient minority and socioeconomic status effects, 137, 138
randomized efficacy studies and, 168
review process, 120-121
study population considerations, 116-117, 137, 138, 168-169
study selection criteria, 118-120
summary and conclusions, 166, 168-171
sustainability of interventions, 170-171
Chronic illness management, guidelines and care protocols, 25, 30, 82, 91-93, 120, 121, 131
anticoagulation, 158
arthritis, 167
asthma, 139
benchmarking, 91-93, 105-107
cardiovascular disease, 150, 160
common features of effective programs, 169
congestive heart failure, 148
diabetes (ADA), 91, 114, 125, 173, 183
heart disease, 16, 109, 138, 141, 148
hypertension, 156
physician commitment to, 32
Chronic illness management, literature review:
description and organization of, 8-9
search process and methods, 10-11
summary tables, 172-241
arthritis, 240-241
asthma, 195-211
cardiovascular disease, 225-239
diabetes, 172-194
Chronic illness management, MCOs versus traditional insurance arrangements, 39-61. *See* Managed care organizations, health status and service utilization comparisons with fee-for-service

Chronic illness management, research issues, 35-36, 255-263
attrition, 131, 138, 151-152, 256
challenges for the future, 260-263
discontinuity of enrollment, 90-91, 93
expanding focus, 259
expanding settings, 257-259
generalizability, 131, 138, 144
improving quality, 256-257
managed care organization recruitment, 257-258
organizational issues, 259
Chronic illness management, use of administrative and medical records data, 66, 89-112
advantages, 103
benchmarking, 91-93, 105-107, 109
cautions and limitations, 103-104
cost and utilization improvement, 95-96, 106-107
enrollment continuity issues, 90-91, 93
general goals of data use, 90
high-risk patient characterization, 99-100, 107, 108
identification of improvement opportunities, 108, 109
provider profiling, 97-99, 108
quality of care assessment, 93-95, 106, 109
simulation (cost-effectiveness models), 107, 109
summary (tables), 105-109
Chronic illness management programs, prevalence in managed care organizations, *See* Managed care organizations, prevalence of chronic illness management programs in
Chrvala, C. A., 4
CIGNA Health Plan, 185
Cintron, G., 146
Clark, G. M., 154
Clark, N. M., 132, 132, 132, 149, 154, 157, 169, 215, 227
Cleland, J. G., 141
Clement, D. G., 52, 57, 60
Cleveland Clinic Foundation, 238
Clinical Resource Management (CRM) system, 224

Clough, J. D., 32
Coats, A. J., 141
Cody, E., 122
Cofer, L. A., 150
Cognitive-behavioral interventions, 163, 215, 227
Cogswell, M. E., 46-47
Cohen, J. L., 164
Cohn, J. N., 138, 141
Colby, C. J., 106
Comprehensive Diabetes Care Service, 182
Computer applications, xi, 120, 121
  anticoagulation, 158
  arthritis, 167
  asthma, 139
  cardiovascular disease, 151, 160
  diabetes, 128, 184
  heart failure, 148
  hypertension, 156
Congestive heart failure (CHF) management, 4, 16-17
  ACE inhibitor use, 115, 138, 141, 144, 214, 223
  at-risk populations, 28
  beta blocker use, 17, 141
  comprehensive management program, 214
  continuous quality improvement initiative, 224
  cost analysis, 217
  disease management programs, 69, 73
  educational interventions, 215-217, 221
  development and implementation of programs, 75, 78
  effective intervention implementation issues, 115
  guidelines, 16, 109, 138, 141, 148
  home-care program, 222
  intervention effectiveness studies, 138, 141-147
    common study features and limitations, 147
    compliance with guidelines, 141
    components of programs (tables), 148-149
    hospital admissions and, 142, 143-144
    hospital-based interventions, 142, 145-146
    memberwide interventions, 142
    non-pharmacological therapies, 141
    pharmacological interventions, 138, 141
    programwide interventions, 143-145
    summary, 146-148
  multidisciplinary interventions, 141-142, 148, 169, 216-219
  nurse-managed interventions, 212-213, 219-221
  pharmacy-based intervention, 223
  quality of care assessment, 109
  service utilization and outcomes, MCOs versus fee-for-service, 54, 58-59
  summary of studies (table), 212-224
Conrad, P., 4
CONSENSUS Trial Study Group, 141
Consumer Reports, 100
Conte, R. R., 154, 159, 235
Continuous quality improvement, 121, 126
  anticoagulation interventions, 159
  arthritis interventions, 167
  asthma interventions, 140, 208-209
  cardiovascular disease interventions, 151-152, 161, 237
  diabetes interventions, 123, 130, 192-194
  heart failure interventions, 149, 224
  hypertension interventions, 157
Cook, K., 154
Cook, S., 127
Coordination of care, 27, 30, 68, 188
  arthritis interventions, 162
  carve-out arrangements and, 35
  open-access plans and, 34
  vendor products and carve-outs, 80
  See also Multidisciplinary teams
Coronary artery disease, 4, 13
Corticosteroids. *See* Inhaled anti-inflammatory medications
Cost and utilization outcomes, 95-96
  asthma interventions, 136-137, 201, 205

Index

congestive heart failure intervention, 217
diabetes interventions, 188, 191, 192
provider profiling, 97-99, 124
Cost-effectiveness models, 100-105, 107
Crabtree, B. F., 122
Creer, T., 132
Criswell, L. A., 57
Cronan, T. A., 109
Cropp, G. J., 132

DaSilva, R. V., 83-84, 86
Databases, 10
Davidson, B. N., 42
Davidson, M. B., 91-93, 105, 114, 122, 123, 130, 131, 183
Davis, C., xii, 68, 70-72
Davis, K. C., 109
Davis, P., 163
de la Sota, A., 132
DeBusk, R. F., 153, 161, 169, 236
Defined contribution plans, 262
Demers, D., 102-103, 107
Der, E., 146
DeVellis, B. M., 164
DeVellis, R. F., 164
DeVries, A., 97-99
Diabetes, 4, 11-12
Diabetes Care Management, 189
Diabetes Care System, 179
Diabetes Control and Complications Trial (DCCT), 12, 83, 114, 122, 171, 188
Diabetes Cooperative Care Clinic (DCCC), 178
Diabetes Electronic Management System (DEMS), 177
Diabetes management, 12-13, 69, 73
American Diabetes Association guidelines, 91, 114, 125, 173, 183
community-based intervention, 187
components of programs (table), 128-130
Comprehensive Diabetes Care Services, 182-183
continuous quality improvement, 192-194
cost-effectiveness models, 102, 107
costs and utilization, 96, 124

identification of study populations, 92-93
development and implementation of programs, 75, 78
effective intervention implementation issues, 114
expenditures, 22
eye examinations, 13, 83, 91-92, 114, 126, 188, 189
foot examinations, 13, 83, 114, 126, 188
HbA1c testing, 12-13, 82, 92, 94, 114, 123-124, 126, 127, 172, 173, 175, 176, 177, 178, 179, 180, 182, 183, 184, 188, 189, 190, 191, 192
health indicators, 125
high-risk patients, 28, 107, 179
identification of opportunities for improvement, 106-107
intervention effectiveness studies, 122-131
  common limitations of reviewed studies, 131
  hospital-based interventions, 126-127
  memberwide interventions, 123-125
  process improvements, 125, 127-128
  programwide interventions, 125-126
  summary, 127
managed care and potential improvements, 31
miniclinics or dedicated days, 122, 129, 193
multidisciplinary care, 122, 128, 169, 174, 178-179, 181, 194
national health care expenditures, 4
nurse case management, 180, 182-184, 194
nutritional interventions, 172, 173
patient characteristics, HMO versus fee-for-service programs, 45
pharmacy-based intervention, 186
practice guidelines, 13, 91-93, 114, 105-106
Project IDEAL, 122, 124, 192-193
quality of care, 94, 106

self-management education and support, 174-175
service utilization and outcomes, MCOs versus fee-for-service, 52-53, 57-58, 60
Staged Diabetes Management (SDM), 82-83, 85, 176, 191
summary of studies (table), 172-194
vendor products, 81-83, 114, 129, 189
Diabetes NetCare, 83, 85, 86, 114, 188
Diabetes Treatment Centers of America, 83, 188
Diehr, P., 42
Dietary interventions, 141, 172, 173, 238
Dietrich, K. A., 13, 83, 114
Digoxin, 16, 141
Diuretic use, 16, 141
Diversified Pharmaceutical Services (DPS), 84, 202
Djkowich, B., 163
Dolovich, J., 132
Domar, A. D., 141
Domurat, E. S., 130, 179
Donahue, J. G., 100, 108
Dowd, B., 43, 44, 47, 60
Dracup, K., 141
Dreyer, N. A., 107, 109
Dreyfus, T., 33
Dropout rates. *See* Attrition
Drug coverage, 25, 90-91
Drug development, 260
Druss, B. G., 50, 55
Duke University Medical Center, 223
Dukes, K. R., 16, 138
Durcanin-Robbins, J. F., 96, 107
Dyslipidemia management, 69, 73, 147, 153
cardiovascular disease interventions, 152-153
care guidelines, 150
intervention program common features, 155
memberwide interventions, 151
nurse-managed intervention, 239
nutritional intervention, 238
program development and implementation, 79
summary of studies (table), 238-239

See also Cardiovascular disease management; Congestive heart failure management

Edelstein, E. L., 122, 127, 130, 181
Educational interventions, 66, 120
anticoagulation, 158, 232
arthritis, 15-16, 162-167, 240
asthma, 132-133, 139, 195-201, 204, 205, 209, 210, 211
cardiovascular diseases, 13, 160
common features of effective programs, 169, 170
diabetes, 122, 128, 174, 186
heart failure, 17, 148, 215-217
hypertension, 156, 225-227
See also Provider education
Effectiveness, of chronic illness management initiatives. *See* Chronic illness management, effectiveness of targeted initiatives
Elderly:
arthritis interventions, 162
health status comparisons, HMOs versus fee-for-service patients, 48
innovative service programs, 70-72
service utilization and outcomes, MCOs versus fee-for-service, 51, 52, 57, 60
trends, 22
Electronic medical records system, 177
Ellenbecker, C. H., 140
Else, B. A., 106
Emergency room visits:
asthma intervention outcomes, 135, 200, 201, 204-205, 211
heart failure intervention outcomes, 143-144, 153, 213-214
See also Hospitalization outcomes
Employee programs, 7, 261-263
access issues for at-risk populations, 28-29
defined contribution plans, 262
diabetes services, 69
elimination of choice, 34
Empowerment, 122
Engelgau, M. M., 106
Ensor, T., 24

Episodes of Care (EOC), 81-82, 114, 189, 208
Epstein, A. M., 50, 56
Epstein, W. V., 56
Etzwiler, D. D., 12, 122
Evidence-based guidelines. *See* Chronic illness management, guidelines and care protocols
Exercise, 141, 236
Expert systems, 120
Eye examinations, 13, 83, 91-92, 114, 126, 188, 189

Fabbri, S. A., 146
Fallon Community Health Plan, 108
Fama, T., 27, 28, 46, 49, 55
The Family Asthma Program, 132
Family PharmaCare Center, Inc., 85
Family Practice Medical Group, Inc., 234
Feagles, L. L., 16, 138
Fee-for-service, comparison with managed care organizations, 39-61. *See* Managed care organizations, health status and service utilization comparisons with fee-for-service
Feigenbaum, P. G., 57
Feldman, R., 43, 44, 47, 60
Feldstein, P. J., 42
Fennell, M., 22
Ferry, D., 146
Financial risk, 28-29, 33-34
Finch, M., 43
Fitzgerald, J. F., 146
Flagstad, M. S., 84
Fletcher Allen Health Care, 102, 107
Follath, F., 141
Foot examinations, 13, 83, 114, 126, 188
Forced expiratory volume, 135-136
Foris, M., 114
Forshee, J. D., 137, 138, 170, 197
Fortuin, N. J., 141
Fowles, Jinnet Briggs, xvi
Fox, H. B., 68
Fox, P. D., 6, 7, 27, 28, 46
Fragmentation of care, 35
Frank, R. G., 42
Frankl, H., 59
Franz, M. J., 116, 125, 130, 131, 172

Freedman, J. A., 146
Fresno Asthma Project (FAP), 117, 210
Friedman, N., 114, 122, 126, 127, 130, 189
Fries, J. F., 164-167, 168, 240
Funke Kupper, A. J., 141

Gabel, J., 24
Gaffrey, S., 24
Garabedian-Ruffalo, S. M., 150, 154
Gatekeeping, 24, 29-30
Gattis, W. A., 149, 223
Geffner, D. L., 122, 130, 185
Generalizability issues, 131, 138, 144
Georgiou, D., 141
Gerber, J. C., 117, 122, 130, 150, 157, 186, 187, 231
Gertler, P., 42
Gheorghiade, M., 141
Gibson, G., 132
Gibson, R., 23, 27
Gilbert, J. A., 1
Gilmet, G. P., 130, 190
Ginsberg, B. H., 12, 82-83, 122, 130, 169, 191
Glasgow, R. E., 12, 122
Glauber, H., x, 96, 106
Gleeson, J. M., 114
Glucose testing. *See* HbA1c testing
Goeppinger, J., 162, 163
Goetsch, M. A., 108
Gold, M. R., 24
Gonzalez, V. M., 164
Goonan, K. J., 137, 140, 208
Gottlieb, L. K., 95, 109
Graff, W. L., 122, 127, 130, 182
Grana, J., 99-100, 108
Gravdal, J. A., 50
Gray, D. B., 115
Gray, D. R., 150
Grazier, K. L., 42
Green, L. W., 132, 153
Greene, A. B., Jr., 140, 211
Greenfield, S., 51, 53, 56, 57
Greineder, D. K., 108, 132, 135, 136, 137, 140, 169, 170, 204-205
Griffin, K. W., 138, 140, 170, 199
Group education, 163

Group Health of Puget Sound, 5, 48, 49, 106, 182, 193, 257
Group Health of Seattle, 164, 240

Haller, V., 58
Hamer, R., 23, 24
Hampson, S. E., 12, 122
Hanchak, N. A.,
Harvard Community Health Plan, 95, 100, 109, 135, 174, 204-205, 208
Hasan, M. M., 115
Hassanein, R., 163
Hatch, M. H., 13, 114
Hawaii Medical Service Association, 105, 106, 107
Hawk, A. D., 13, 83, 114
Hawley, D. J., 15, 162, 163, 164
Hawthorne, M. H., 141
Hayati, F., 115
HbA1c testing, 12-13, 82, 92, 94, 114, 123-124, 126, 127, 172, 173, 175, 176, 177, 178, 179, 180, 182, 183, 184, 188, 189, 190, 191, 192
Health Belief Model, 226
Health Care Financing Administration, 3
Health maintenance organizations (HMOs), x, 1. *See* Managed care organizations
Health Net, 91, 93, 106, 107, 108, 114, 126, 184
Health Partners (or HealthPartners), 123, 151, 192, 257
Health-related quality of life, asthma interventions and, 134. *See also* Quality of life
Health Services Advisory Group, Inc., 94
HealthStar, 10
HealthSystem Minnesota, 229
Healthtrac, 164, 240
Healy, J. M., Jr., 137
Heart disease. *See* Cardiovascular disease management; Congestive heart failure management
Hedblom, E. C., 96
HEDIS, 31, 91, 113
Heidenreich, P. A., 146
Heinen, L., 130, 191
Hellinger, F. J., 41

Henderson, W. G., 146
Hendricson, W. D., 133
Hennelly, V. D., 42
Hernandez, E., 146
Hershey Medical Center, 219
Heywood, J. T., 146
High-risk patients or populations, 99-100
 access issues, 28-29, 33
 common features of effective programs, 169
 diabetes intervention, 179
 intervention effectiveness considerations, 117-118, 137
 patient characterization, 107
Hillman, A. L., 33
Hillson, S., 97-99
Himmel, J. K., 163
Hindi-Alexander, M. C., 132
Hindmarsh, M., x
Hirano, P. C., 15, 155, 162
HMO Workgroup, 35
Hoechst Marion Roussel, 24, 187
Hofer, T. P., 53, 58
Hoffman, C., 3, 22
Holman, H. R., 56, 163, 164
Home visits, 129, 140
 anticoagulation interventions, 158
 arthritis interventions, 167
 asthma interventions, 140, 203
 cardiovascular disease interventions, 160, 225
 diabetes interventions, 129
 heart failure interventions, 148, 222
 hypertension interventions, 156
Homer, C. J., 14, 132
Honda, G. D., 59
Horowitz, M., 137
Hospital-based studies, 119, 126-127
 cardiovascular disease interventions, 153-154
 congestive heart failure, 142, 145-146
Hospitalization outcomes, 83, 135, 204-206, 208
 asthma interventions and, 196, 201, 202, 211
 cardiovascular disease interventions and, 153
 diabetes interventions and, 179, 188
 disease management programs and, 84

heart disease interventions and, 142, 143-144, 213-214, 216, 220-221
MCO members versus fee-for-service participants, 50, 58
See also Emergency room visits
Howell, T., 14, 137
Hughes, G. W., 137
Hurley, R., 24
Hydralazine isosorbide dinitrate, 16, 141
Hypercholesterolemia. *See* Dyslipidemia management
Hypertension management, 69, 73, 147, 151-157
 educational interventions, 225-227
 guidelines, 150
 hospital-based interventions, 153
 intervention program common features, 155
 intervention program components, 156-157
 memberwide interventions, 151-152
 nurse-managed interventions, 229-230
 patient characteristics, HMO versus fee-for-service programs, 45
 program development and implementation, 79
 provider training initiatives, 228
 quality of care studies, 94
 service utilization and outcomes, MCOs versus fee-for-service, 50-51, 56, 60
 summary of studies (table), 225-231
 See also Cardiovascular disease management

IDEAL, 122, 124, 192-193
In Control, 175
Independent physician associations (IPAs), x, 23, 32-34, 258
 asthma intervention outcomes, 202
Information technologies, 261
Ingram, R. E., 163
Inhaled anti-inflammatory medications, 84, 93, 115, 131-133, 195, 197, 202, 204
Innovative or effective programs, 70-72
INSPIRE, 197

Institute for Clinical Systems Improvement (ICSI), 138, 141, 152
Institute of Medicine, 3
Insulin dependent diabetes mellitus (IDDM), 11-12. *See* Diabetes management
Integrated Therapeutics Group (ITG), 84, 197, 202
International Diabetes Center, 81, 82, 191
Internet, 261
InterStudy, 24, 25, 72-79, 86
Ireys, H. T., 58

Jackson, C., 42
Jacksonville Health Care Group, 125, 180
Jacobs, R., 30-31, 33, 150
Jacobs, S. C., 141
Jatulis, D. E., 93, 107
Jennings, B., 3
Jennison, K., 56
Jensen, G., 24
Jewish Hospital, 115, 216-217
Joint National Committee on Detection, Evaluation, and Treatment of High Blood Pressure, 147
Joint pain, 51-52, 56
Jones, P. K., 132, 153, 157, 226
Jones, S. L., 132, 154
Jones, T., 14, 137
Jordan, H. S., 107, 137
Joshi, 130, 169, 194
Joslin Diabetes Center, 231
Journals, 10
Juba, D. A., 42
Judd, B. J., 163

Kaiser Health Plans, 5
Kaiser Permanente:
 Baltimore, 205
 Colorado, 98, 108, 109
 New York, 206
 Northern California, 51, 92, 106, 107, 109, 135-136, 144, 153, 178, 179, 196, 200, 210, 213, 214, 236, 257
 Northwest, 96, 107, 108, 109, 199
 Southern California, 54, 135, 136, 186, 201, 204

Kane, R., 22, 70
Kaplan, D. L., 132
Kaplan, M., 132
Kaplan, R. M., 163
Karp, D., 154
Katz, B. P., 146
Katz, J., 132, 154
Keefe, F. J., 163
Kehoe, W. A., 154
Kent, M. J., 114
Kerr, E., 7
Klein, W., 141
Klemchuk, H., 141
Koplan, J. P., 4, 46-47
Kosinski, M., 48
Kotses, H., 132
Kowal, C. E., 133, 137, 140, 195
Kraines, R. G., 164
Krantz, 54
Kravitz, R. L., 44-45, 47
Kronick, R., 33
Kropfelder, L., 135, 137, 140, 205
Kurata, J. H., 59

La Forge, R., 154, 161, 239
Lake, T., 24
Laliberte, L., 22
Lanes, S. F., 107, 109
Lanza, L. L., 109
Laris, B. A., 164
Lasater, M., 142, 146, 149, 221
Lasker, R. D., 12, 122
Laurent, D. D., 15, 155, 164
Lave, J. R., 42
Laville, E. A., 162
Leake, B., 133
Lee, D., 141
Lee, P. P., 53, 58
Legacy 2000, 187, 231
Legorreta, A. P., 91-93, 105, 107, 108, 115, 130, 169, 184
Lehigh Valley Hospital, 219
Leong, A. B., 101-102
Leong, D., 16, 138
Leung, K. M., 115
Levin, R., 58
Levine, D. M., 153
Lewis, B. E., 107

Lewis, C. E., 132, 135, 136, 138, 140, 170, 201
Lewis, M. A., 132
Lieu, T. A., 14, 101-102, 108, 109, 132
Life expectancy, 22
Linares, E., 146
Lindroth, Y., 163-164
Lipid management. *See* Dyslipidemia management
Lipid Management Clinic, 238
Lipid monitoring, 13, 126, 189
Liston, D., 24
Literature review methodology. *See* Chronic illness management, literature review
Liu, G., 122
Livingston, J. M., 108
Living With Asthma, 132
Loane, K. C., 132
Lodhia, H., 154
Long, S. H., 42
Lorig, K., 15, 155, 162, 163, 164
Lorish, C. D., 163
Lousberg, T. R., 109
Lovelace Health System, 81, 106, 114, 127, 189, 208, 259
Lowe, J. C., 163
Lozano, P., 14, 132
Lubeck, D., 51, 56, 164
Lucas, S., 133
Ludwig-Beymer, P., 140, 211
Luft, H., 5
Luther, P., 115

MacKenzie, E. J., 132
MacKinnon, N. J., 84
Maiman, L. A., 132, 141
Managed care, ix-x
 current debate, 30-35
 defining, 5-7
 early concerns, 26-30, 40
 research issues, 35-36. *See also* Chronic illness management, research issues
 trends, 23-26
Managed care organizations (MCOs):
 access issues for at-risk populations, 28-29, 33
 backlash against, 2

defining, 5-7
discussion of findings, 59-61
factors affecting health plan choice, 40-41
information technology use, 261
insurance function, 7
Medicare and Medicaid contracts, 25-26
Medicare market penetration, 67
multi-organizational interactions, x-xi, 66-67
new drug development and, 260
organizational issues of chronic care, 259
performance standards, 31
physician membership issues, x-xi
policy issues and debates, 2
potential for improvement over usual care, 27-28, 30-31
potential limitations and shortcomings, 28-30, 32-35
recruitment as study participants, 257-258
reimbursement for nonmedical services, 30
specialization and "carve-out" arrangements, 35
trends, 1, 23-25, 66-67
Managed care organizations, chronic illness management programs. *See* Chronic illness management
Managed care organizations, effectiveness of specific programs. *See* Chronic illness management, effectiveness of targeted initiatives
Managed care organizations, health status and service utilization comparisons with fee-for-service, 39-61
health status and enrollment, MCOs versus comparison groups, 43-47
health status and health plan choice studies, 40-43
research questions, 61
service utilization and health status outcomes, 47-59
congestive heart failure, 54, 58-59
diabetes, 52-53, 57-58, 60
elderly patients, 51, 52, 57, 60
general chronic illness, 48, 49-50, 55
hypertension, 50-51, 56, 60
joint pain/rheumatitis/osteoporosis, 51-52, 56-57
peptic ulcer, 54, 59
Managed care organizations, prevalence of chronic illness management programs in, 65-88, 170
carve-outs. *See* Carve-out arrangement
development and implementation, 74-79
general information lack, 86-87
HMO market penetration and, 73
HMO size and, 74
innovative service programs, 70-72
InterStudy survey, 72-79, 86
multiple disease services, 74
small-scale studies, 68-70
vendor products. *See* Vendor products
Wagner et al. study, 70-72, 86
Managed care organizations, use of administrative and medical records data. *See* Chronic illness management, use of administrative and medical records data
Managed indemnity plans, 23, 24
Mandle, C. L., 141
Mangotich, M., 56
Marshall, C. L., 94, 106
Martin, D. K., 146
Martin, D. P., 42
Martin, T. L., 92-93, 105, 114
Massie, B. M., 146
Mayo Clinic, 177, 230
Mazonson, P. D., 164
Mazze, R. S., 12, 82, 122, 130, 169, 191
Mazzuca, S. A., 12, 122, 164
McCallian, D. J., 84-85
McCombs, J. S., 122
McCredie, M., 163-164
McCulloch, D. K., x, 12, 122
McDermott, P. D., 99-100
McGhan, S., 132
McGuire, T. G., 42
McIntyre, K. M., 150
McNabb, W. L., 127, 130, 131, 133, 137, 138, 140, 170, 173, 175, 200

McNeil, B. J., 56
McShane, D. J., 164-167
Mechanic, D., 29-30, 33, 34
Medicaid, 25-26, 54, 207
Medical Nutrition Therapy (MNT), 172
Medical Outcomes Study, 44, 47, 49, 50, 51, 53, 56, 57
Medical record keeping, 104, 177. *See also* Chronic illness management, use of administrative and medical records data
Medical University of South Carolina, 221
Medicare, 25, 52, 67
  drug coverage, 91
  intervention effectiveness assessment issues, 144
  quality of care issues, 94
MedImpact Pharmaceutical Management, Inc., 83
Medline, 10, 119
Meenan, R. F., 109
Memberwide disease management approaches, 117
  asthma, 133-134
  cardiovascular disease, 151-152
  congestive heart failure, 142
  diabetes, 123-125
Mendoza, G. R., 101-102
Mental illness, 5
Merrill, J., 42
Mesch-Beatty, K., 84
Metered dose inhalers (MDIs), 115
Mid Atlantic Medical Services, 197
Mid-Peninsula Health Service, 51, 56
Millennium Healthcare, 187, 231
Miller-Kovach, K., 154
Miniclinics, 121
  asthma, 139
  arthritis, 167
  cardiovascular disease, 160
  common features of effective programs, 169
  diabetes, 122, 129, 193
  heart failure, 148
Minnesota Department of Health, 123, 192
Minorities, 137, 138
Mitchell, I., 132

Model for Effective Chronic Illness Care, 71
Moe, E. L., 136, 137, 140, 199
Monica, E. D., 142, 146
Morgan, L., 164
Morgan, T., 141
Morisky, D. E., 153
Morrisey, M., 24
Mullen, P. D., 162
Multidisciplinary teams, xi, 121
  anticoagulation interventions, 158
  arthritis interventions, 165, 167, 241
  asthma interventions, 139
  cardiovascular disease interventions, 160
  diabetes interventions, 122, 128, 169, 174, 178-179, 181, 194
  heart disease interventions, 141-142, 148, 169, 216-219
  hypertension interventions, 156, 230
  lipid management intervention, 239
MULTIFIT, 144, 213
Multiple chronic illnesses, 257
Murphy, D. M., 127
Murphy, R., 141

Nangle, M., 154, 237
National Asthma Education and Prevention (NAEP) program (NIH), 131-132, 134
National Asthma Education Project (NAEP), 93
National Cholesterol Education Project (NCEP), 147, 238
National Committee for Quality Assurance (NCQA), 31, 67, 91
National Council of State Legislatures, 6
National Health Insurance Experiment, 49
National Health Interview Survey, 46, 49, 162
National Heart, Lung, and Blood Institute, 16, 84, 133
National Medical Expenditure Survey, 3, 45
Nelson, D., 46-47
Nelson, E. C., 50, 60-61
Nestor, A., 107

Index

Networks, x
Neuberger, G. B., 163
Newacheck, P. W., 68
Nichols, G. A., x
Nielson, N., 154
Nolan, S., 14, 132
Non-insulin dependent diabetes mellitus (NIDDM), 12
   identification of study populations, 92-93
   weight-loss program, 173
   See Diabetes management
Nurse case management, 71, 121, 179
   anticoagulation interventions, 158
   asthma interventions, 139, 203, 205
   cardiovascular disease interventions, 160
   congestive heart failure interventions, 144, 213, 218-220
   diabetes management, 128, 180, 182-184, 194
   heart failure interventions, 148
   hypertension interventions, 156
Nurse education. *See* Provider education
Nurse home visits. *See* Home visits
Nutritional interventions, 125, 172, 173, 238
Nyman, J. A., 97-99, 108

O'Brien, K. P., 14, 132
O'Connor, P. J., 122, 123, 124, 127, 130, 150-152, 169, 192, 228
Oddone, E. Z., 146
O'Leary, A., 163
Olesen, K. H., 141
Open-access plans, 24, 34
Open Airways, 132, 199
Osborne, M. L., 105, 107
Ossorio, R. C., 91-93, 114, 123
Osteoarthritis, 15, 155. *See* Arthritis management
Osteoporosis, 51, 56
   disease management programs, 69, 73
   program development and implementation, 79
Outcomes evaluation. *See* Chronic illness management, effectiveness of targeted initiatives; specific chronic illnesses, interventions

Pacala, J., 70
Packer, M., 141
Pai, R., 146
Park Nicollet Institute, xvi
Park Nicollet Medical Center, 151, 165, 229, 241
Parker, J. C., 163
Parks, P., 132
Parmley, W. W., 141
Partners-in-Care, 219
Pastor, M., 14, 137
Patient education, See Educational interventions
Patient empowerment, 122
Patient-level interventions, 120
   anticoagulation, 158
   arthritis, 167
   asthma, 139
   cardiovascular disease, 160, 161
   diabetes, 128
   hypertension, 156
Patient recruitment, 71
Patient satisfaction, 144, 171
Patterson, J. H., 141
Paul, S., 142, 146, 149, 221
Peak-flow meters (PFMs), 115, 132, 197, 199
Pelletier, K. R., 115
Penn State Geisinger Health System, 219
Peptic ulcer, 54, 59, 69, 73, 79
Performance standards, 31
Peters, A. L., 91-93, 105, 115, 122, 125, 130, 131, 182, 183
Peterson, C. R., 84
Peterson, M. G., 164
Petitti, D. B., x
Pfeffer, M. A., 141
Pharmaceutical development, 260
Pharmacist in Health Failure Assessment Recommendation and Monitoring (PHARM), 223
Pharmacy-based interventions, 121
   anticoagulation, 158, 233-236
   arthritis, 167

asthma, 85, 139
cardiovascular disease, 155, 160
diabetes, 122, 129, 186
heart failure, 148, 223
hypertension, 156
Pharmacy Benefits Managers (PBMs), 81
Pharmacy claims data, 92-93
Pheley, A. M., 151, 157, 169, 229
Phillips, R. S., 56
Physician choice, ix
Physician profiling, 83-84, 97-99, 108, 121
  arthritis interventions, 167
  asthma interventions, 139
  cardiovascular disease interventions, 160
  diabetes interventions, 128
  heart failure interventions, 148
Physicians
  acceptance of vendor products, 86
  compliance with managed care treatment guidelines, 32
  contractual relationships with multiple managed care organizations, x, 66-67
  financial risk, 34
  gatekeeping for specialist services, 24, 29-30
  managed care organizations influence on decision making, 66-67
  satisfaction, 144
  support for chronic illness management initiatives, 66-67
Platt, R., 108
Plaut, T. F., 14, 137, 140, 203, 206
Practice redesign, 120
Preferred provider organizations (PPOs), x, 23-24, 32-34, 258
  chronic disease programs, 77
  enrollment choice studies, 41
Prescription drug coverage, 25, 90-91
Preston, J. A., 51, 52, 56, 57, 58, 60
Preston, S., 99-100
Price, M. J., x
Priestley, D., 164
Primary physicians, gatekeeping for specialist services, 24, 29-30
PrimeCare, 114, 126, 189
Principle Health Care, 203

Profitability issues, 32-33
Programwide disease management approaches, 117
  arthritis interventions, 164-166
  asthma interventions, 134-137
  cardiovascular disease interventions, 152-153
  congestive heart failure interventions, 143-145
  diabetes interventions, 125-126
Project IDEAL, 122, 124, 192-193
Pronk, N. P., 123, 130, 192
Proudlock, M., 132
Provider education:
  anticoagulation, 158
  arthritis, 167
  asthma, 139, 197, 203
  cardiovascular disease, 160
  diabetes, 128, 178
  heart failure, 148
  hypertension, 156, 228
Provider-level interventions, 121
Provider profiling, 97-99, 108
Prudential Health Care, 46, 109, 180
Public/private partnerships, 121
  anticoagulation interventions, 159
  arthritis interventions, 167
  asthma management, 84, 140
  cardiovascular disease interventions, 161
  diabetes management, 129
  hypertension interventions, 157
Public/private partnerships, 140
Pugh, L. C., 142, 146, 149, 219
Purcaro, A., 141

Quality assurance, 121, 31
  anticoagulation interventions, 159
  arthritis interventions, 167
  asthma interventions, 140
  benchmarking, 91-93
  diabetes interventions, 130
  heart failure interventions, 149
  hypertension interventions, 157
Quality improvement, continuous. *See* Continuous quality improvement
Quality Improvement Project, 209
Quality of life outcomes, 171

Index   281

asthma intervention, 134, 197, 202
cardiovascular health intervention, 237
congestive heart failure intervention,
    215, 217
diabetes intervention, 183
disease management program, 84
hypertension intervention, 227
Quality Screening Management (QSM),
    191
Quandt, C. M., 154
Quesenberry, C. P., 101-102
Quickel, K. E., Jr., 4, 22, 30, 31
Quinn, M. T., 127

Rachelefsky, G., 132
Radensky, P. W., 109
RAND National Health Insurance
    Experiment, 48
Randomized efficacy trials, 113-114
Ray, G. T., 106
Retchin, S. M., 51, 52, 56, 57
Retinal exams, 91-92, 114, 126, 184
Reuter, J., 42
Rheumatitis, 51-52, 56
Rheumatoid arthritis, 15, 155, 162. *See
    also* Arthritis management
Rice, D., 3, 22
Rich, M. W., 115, 141, 142, 149, 216-217
Richards, W., 133
Richardson, W. C., 42
Rippey, R. M., 164
Robinson, J., 7
Rodriguez, D. J., 114
Roethel, C. R., 13, 114
Rogers, W., 48, 56
Rognehaugh, R., 6
Rosenstein, A. H., 149, 224
Rosenstock, I. M., 12, 122
Rosiello, R. A., 107
Rospond, R. M., 154
Rossiter, L. F., 41
Rothenberg, R. B., 4
Rothfield, N., 164
Rubin, R. J., 13, 83, 85, 86, 114, 122, 130,
    169, 188
Ruffalo, R. L., 150
Ruggerio, C., 146
Rupp, M. T., 84-85

Sadur, C. N., 130, 178
St. Francis Hospital and Medical Center,
    177
St. Luke's Hospital, 226, 237
St. Paul Children's Hospital, 198
Salem-Schatz, S., 95, 109
Salkever, D. S., 153
San Diego Cardiac Center Medical
    Group, 239
San Francisco General Hospital, 235
San Joaquin Valley Health Consortium,
    210
Sandy, L. G., 23, 27
Satisfaction outcomes, 55, 144, 171
Sauter, S. V., 164
Sax, M. J., 150
Scamagas, P., 137
Scanlon, D. P., 42
Schaefer, J., xii, 68, 70-72
Schauffler, H., 69
Schlesinger, M., 27, 29-30, 33, 34, 55
Schmitt, D. D., 154
Schnatz, J. D., 122
Schned, E. S., 165-167, 241
Schultz, J. F., 157, 230
Schupp, K., 154
Scocco, V., 141
Scripps Health Chronic Care Clinic, 212
Seabrook, G. R., 154, 159, 232
Seelbinder, J. S., 142, 146, 149, 218
Selby, J. V., 92-93, 105, 106, 114
Seleznick, M., 164
Self, T., 14, 132
Self-management education. *See*
    Educational interventions
Self-reported measures, 46
Sennett, C., 31
Service Line Management, 237
Settle, R. F., 42
Shaddy, J., 42
Shah, N. B., 146
Sharfstein, S., 4
Shatin, D., 53, 58
Shearn, M. A., 56
Sheehan, T. J., 164
Sheffer, A. L., 107
Sheth, K. K., 84-85
Shields, M. C., 138, 140, 170, 199
Shoor, S., 163

Short, P. F., 42
Shulkin, D., 33, 67
Sigurd, B., 141
Simulation models, 100-105
Singer, D. L., 130, 174
Sloss, E. M., 48, 49
Smith, D. M., 146
Smith, K. V., 163
Smith, L. E., 146
Smith, S. A., 127, 130, 177
Smoking-cessation programs, 153, 236
Snyder, S. E., 132, 133
Socioeconomic status effects, 137, 138
Sociology, 4
Sodium-restricted diet, 141
Sofaer, S., 42
Solberg, L. I., 122, 123, 124, 130, 170, 193
SOLVD Investigators, 141
Sorel, M. E., 101-102
Specialist services or referrals:
　anticoagulation interventions, 159
　arthritis interventions, 167
　asthma interventions, 140
　cardiovascular disease interventions, 161
　cost and utilization studies, 98
　diabetes interventions, 129
　gatekeeping, 24, 29-30
　heart failure interventions, 149
　hypertension interventions, 156
　open-access approach, 24, 34
Sperrl-Hillen, J., x
Staged Diabetes Management (SDM), 82-83, 85, 176, 191
Stegall, M. H., 57
Stempel, D. A., 96, 107
Stevens, M. A., 132, 137, 140, 206
Stewart, D. L., 117, 130, 150, 157, 187, 231
Stoner, T., 97-99
Strauss, G. D., 163
Strokes, 150
Sturm, L. L., 96
Substance abuse, 5
Sullivan, M. J., 141
Sullivan, S., 14, 132, 134
Sung, H. Y., 3, 22
Svensk, U., 1

System-based approaches, 1, 31, 121
Systemic lupus erythematosus, 155

Taggart, V. S., 133
Take Pride, 227
Tan, M. H., 82-83, 169
Taniguchi, J., 163
Tarlov, A. R., 48, 56
Taylor, A. K., 42, 45-46
Terry, K., 127, 140, 189, 208
Texas Heart Institute, 237
Thomas, T., 55, 154
Thorp, F. K., 127
Toledo Hospital, 220
Topol, E. J., 141
Topp, R., 145, 149, 220
Toscano, James V., xvi
Towne, J. B., 154
Traill, T. A., 141
Trubitt, M. J., 140, 207
Tucker, D., 145
Tufts University, 176
Turner, R. A., 163
Type 1 diabetes, 11-12. *See* Diabetes management; Insulin dependent diabetes mellitus
Type 2 diabetes, 12. *See* Diabetes management; Non-insulin dependent diabetes mellitus

U-Care, 84
Udvarhelyi, I. S., 51, 56
United Health Care (or United HealthCare), 6, 54, 96, 98, 106, 108, 191, 207
University of Pennsylvania, 194, 259
University of Virginia, 232
Urden, L. D., 142, 146, 149, 219
Uretsky, B. F., 141

Vendor products, 80-86, 121
　anticoagulation interventions, 159
　arthritis interventions, 167
　asthma interventions, 81, 83-86, 140
　cardiovascular disease interventions, 161

Index 283

diabetes interventions, 81-83, 114, 129, 189
Episodes of Care (EOC), 81-82, 114, 189, 208
heart failure interventions, 149
health outcomes and costs, 85
hypertension interventions, 157
physician acceptance of, 86
use with multiple diseases, 81-82
Venner, G. H., 142, 146, 149, 218
Veterans' Administration, 119, 146, 154
Vinicor, 23
Vistnes, J. P., 45-46
Vollmer, W. M., 107, 108
von Korff, M., x, xii, 23, 68, 70-72, 86, 114
Votaw, R. G., 164

Waagstein, F., 141
Wagner, E. H., x, xi, xii, 12, 23, 25, 27, 32, 68, 70-72, 86, 114, 115, 119-121, 123, 130, 170, 193
Walker, A. M., 107, 109
Walsh, S., 14, 137
Ward, M. M., 52
Ware, J. E.., Jr., 48, 49
Washburne, W. F., 115
Washington University Medical Center, 115, 216-217
Web sites, 261
Weber, C., 145
Wee Wheezers, 136, 198
Weight-loss program, 173
Weinberger, M., 146
Weiss, S. T., 108
Weiss-Harrison, A., 132, 137, 140, 206
Welch, W. P., 42

Wennevold, A., 141
Wesolowski, W., 13, 114
West, J. A., 142, 144, 149, 169, 170, 213
Westley, C. R., 98-99, 108
Wetstone, S. L., 164
Wheeler, D. A., 115
Wheezers Anonymous, 132
Whight, C., 141
White, L. A., 46
Wicks, L. B., 68
Wilensky, G. R., 41
Wilkes, R. M., 16, 138, 141, 142-144, 149, 169, 214
Williamson, J., 122
Wilson, M., 141
Wilson, S. R., 117, 133, 135, 136, 137, 138, 140, 170, 196, 198, 210
Wilson-Pessano, S. R., 133, 137, 140, 169, 196
Wilt, V. M., 159, 234
Winder, J. A., 132
Wittenberg, C., 115
Wood, K., 34
Wrightson, C. W., Jr., 42

Yelin, E. H., 52, 56, 57
Yood, R. A., 109
You Can Control Asthma, 133
Young, L. D., 163, 141

Zazzali, J. L., 137
Zeiger, R. S., 135, 137, 170, 204, 140
Zeller, M., 154
Zhang, D., 92-93, 105, 106, 114
Zhou, Z., 33
Zuckerman, A. E., 133

About the Authors

Jon B. Christianson, PhD, is an economist with extensive research and teaching experience in the financing and delivery of medical care. He has published in the areas of managed care, rural health care, mental health care, and care process improvement, and he has collaborated with health care providers in a variety of practice settings to evaluate new treatment approaches. He received a Ph.D. degree from the University of Wisconsin-Madison and currently is on the faculty of the Carlson School of Management at the University of Minnesota, where he is the James A. Hamilton Chair in Health Policy and Management. He serves on a number of different editorial boards and scientific advisory panels and directs the Center for the Study of Healthcare Management in the Department of Healthcare Management at the Carlson School.

Aylin Altan Riedel holds a PhD in health services research from the University of Minnesota (2000). At the time this manuscript was developed, she was a researcher in the Health Research Center at the Park Nicollet Institute. She is currently a senior research analyst at Ingenix Pharmaceutical Services. Her research interests focus on health outcomes for individuals with chronic illness, with special focus on how the organization of care delivery, self-management strategies, and socioeconomic factors interact to affect outcomes for these patients.

David J. Abelson, M.D., is chair of the Institute for Clinical Systems Improvement (ICSI) and medical director, information management and care improvements, Park Nicollet Clinic and Methodist Hospital in St. Louis Park, Minnesota. He was named guideline implementation leader in 1994 and, in that role, designed and managed support to implement 40 ICSI clinical guidelines. He also designed and managed integration of ambulatory clinical guidelines and hospital pathways as part of a program called Supporting Best Care. He earned a medical degree from the University of Minnesota in 1976 and completed an internship and residency in medicine there in 1979. He is a member of several professional organizations, including the American Board of Internal Medicine, the American Medical Association, the American Medical Informatics Association, and the Healthcare Information and Management Systems Society. He is a frequent speaker at national medical forums and symposiums. He has published numerous articles in medical journals and is the author of the book *Take Charge of Your Health*.

Richard L. Hamer is director of InterStudy Publications, a Minneapolis-based health care research and information company. In addition to having responsibility for general management and organizational development, he directs and supervises personnel engaged in InterStudy's primary research of select managed care and health care quality-management topics. He has previous experience in corporate health maintenance programs and in financial and management consulting for health and human services organizations. He received a BS from the University of Minnesota and an MA from the University of Toronto.

David J. Knutson is director of health systems studies at the Park Nicollet Institute for Research and Education in Minneapolis. He directs research on health policy, health economics, and managed care. He also holds adjunct faculty appointments at the University of Minnesota. Before entering the field of research, he spent many years in health care administration. Most recently, he held the positions of director of research and development and senior director of provider network management for MedCenters Health Plan, a Twin Cities health maintenance organization (HMO), and for Aetna Health Plans. His responsibilities included new HMO development, provider contracting, and product management. His current research focuses on developing and evaluating risk-based payment methods, on measuring and using information on health plan quality for purchasing, and on the cost-effectiveness of clinical care. He has published a number of scientific and policy-related articles and co-authored a recently published book on management of chronic illness.

Ruth A. Taylor is the coordinator of the Center for the Study of Healthcare Management at the Carlson School of Management, University of Minnesota. She earned a bachelor's degree from Valparaiso University. She has extensive experience in program implementation, project management of studies of chronic illness-management initiatives in clinical settings, and coordination of both national and local outcomes studies. She is a member of an Institutional Review Board (IRB) for the protection of human subjects in research and sits on the Advisory Committee for a local health care system's three IRBs. She has collaborated with Dr. Christianson on several projects and publications focusing on the management of chronic illness in health care organizations.